# herbal
## home doctor

# herbal
# home doctor

herbal, homeopathic and ayurvedic remedies – achieving
vital whole health from nature's medicine chest

Robin Hayfield, Sue Hawkey,
Sally Morning star

HERMES
HOUSE

This edition is published by Hermes House

Hermes House is an imprint of Anness Publishing Ltd
Hermes House, 88–89 Blackfriars Road, London SE1 8HA
tel. 020 7401 2077; fax 020 7633 9499; info@anness.com

A CIP catalogue record for this book is available from the British Library.

Publisher: Joanna Lorenz
Managing Editor: Helen Sudell
Project Editor: Emma Gray
Additional text by: Stephanie Donaldson, Jessica Houdret and Mark Evans
Designer: Balley Design Associates; Illustrator: Giovanna Pierce
Photographers: Don Last, John Freeman and Michelle Garrett
Production Controller: Claire Rae

Previously published as *Natural Healing*

1 3 5 7 9 10 8 6 4 2

# contents

# natural healing introduction

One of the key issues today is knowing exactly how to look after yourself, and that does not just mean steering clear of all kinds of excesses that are known to be bad for you, such as coffee, alcohol and stress. It means knowing the many subtle and sophisticated ways in which the body works, which are largely ignored by conventional medicine. Knowing, for example, how the deft use of herbalism can quickly help you to revive after a tiring, difficult day, how using homeopathy can bolster your body's well-being and how the ancient Indian healing technique, Ayurveda, can help you tackle all kinds of illnesses holistically. using diet, colours, gems and crystals.

# healing naturally

Health is the most natural state of being. The root of the word "health" is related not only to "healing" but also to "wholeness", and it is precisely that sense of wholeness and of being in tune – physically, mentally and spiritually – that makes you feel your best. In recent years there has been a massive revival of interest in natural therapies, both in recognition of their tremendous value and as a move away from the impersonal approach and unwelcome side-effects of conventional medicine. Much of this is simply because natural therapists often take more time to get to know the whole person, the whole you, and acknowledge the wider aspects of health. The gentle, natural remedies that they employ have been tried and tested over centuries, and can be effective not just in returning your system to normal when you are ill, but as a means of optimizing your well-being and general state of health.

It is easy to think of medicine only as a crisis treatment for when you are sick, and this is the basis of most ordinary medical practice. Many people neglect their general health until they become ill and then turn to medicine for the cure. Getting the most out of life means looking after yourself every day and not just trying to cure illness when it arrives. This means boosting your own natural energies to keep yourself in good shape. A healthy body is far less likely to suffer setbacks, and if they do happen it is more likely to cure itself, quickly and completely. Being healthy means being in touch with every part of your being and situation; understanding your strengths and weaknesses and staying true to your character and abilities. One of the strengths of natural therapies is the value they place in early, self-help treatment; in this way the extent of an infection, bacterial or viral, is minimized, and the load that is placed on the immune system is reduced to the barest minimum.

Natural therapies are particularly successful in countering the effects of stress on the body and mind, thus actually helping to reduce the likelihood of illness. Stress is recognized as a major factor affecting health in modern society, but what is little

# healing  strengthening
# invigorating

understood are the physiological reasons why stress does have such a marked impact on our overall health. Stress re-apportions the supply of blood and nerve energy to different

areas, increasing the activity of certain organs and reducing the work of others. In prolonged situations of stress, many functions, vital for everyday health, can be neglected, and over a period of time, the body will begin to suffer and show signs of strain, at which point ill-health will appear, or a weakened condition will worsen. The increasing pace and complexity of modern life, juggling the demands of work and family, places great burdens on the body and it is vital to redress the balance before the strain becomes too great and begins to affect our health. By taking some simple and pleasurable steps to restore

and enhance your own vital energy, you can actively reduce the impact of the worries that you encounter in daily life. Principally, rest is required and attention must be paid to the specific symptoms that you suffer, and this is where this book will offer valuable advice. It is important to try not to spend time worrying about not feeling well, or feeling pressurized, but try and access the nervous energy that comes with stress and use it as a motivational tool to change the things that are affecting your health.

The key to the success of most holistic therapies is that they take into account the mental, emotional and spiritual well-being of a person, as well as the physical aspects of health. Holistic therapies recognize that physical symptoms, such as headaches and stomach upsets, and emotional ones, such as depression, can interweave to create more serious disease.

In order to help reduce the impact of stress on your whole system, you need to find ways both to avoid becoming stressed in the first place, and to release the changes that occur internally. Looking after yourself with a nourishing diet and regular exercise will help you feel better and more able to cope with issues that you really cannot avoid.

The traditions of natural medicine are based on a vast accumulation of practical knowledge. Herbal remedies are almost certainly the most popular and most easily understood method of self-help treatment. The medicines given are all extracted from plants, and as with many other complementary treatments they may also be combined with other general health advice. Herbalism is excellent for minor complaints and such problems as anxiety, indigestion and hangovers; the problems can be simply and easily treated using herbal cures that are easy to make. Infusions, which are rather like herb teas, are a delicious and safe way to take medicinal herbs. Herbs may also be taken as tinctures or syrups. Scented herbal baths are a real pleasure and remarkably effective for treating certain complaints. Herbal remedies will alleviate many common

symptoms, and there are numerous simple herbal recipes in this book that can be used.

Illnesses can also be treated with homeopathic remedies which you can administer yourself. Homeopathy was discovered in the 18th century by Samuel Hahnemann who began the experiments that led to the development and principles of the modern therapy. In homeopathy, symptoms are seen not as the negative effects of illness, but as the attempts of the individual to resist disease. Hence a remedy that produces the symptoms of a particular illness in a healthy person is administered in minute doses to a person with those symptoms. Homeopaths describe this as treating "like with like". Since the remedies are given in such minute doses, it is surmised that they

are acting not on the physical body, but on the surrounding energies of the body. This encourages and supports the body's own self-healing mechanisms, enabling it to combat the disease effectively and in a natural manner that is controlled by the body itself.

Traditional healing therapies have evolved in most cultures in the East and in the West. The ancient Indian system of Ayurveda is thought to be one of the oldest healing disciplines in the world. Like much of Eastern ideology, it involves energy: it views all parts of the human body as being interconnected and infused with vital forces, which are constantly revitalizing themselves. The body is not just regarded as an empty vessel into which you pour the

herbalism
homeopathy
ayurveda

wholeness gentleness
healing invigorating soothing energizing

remedies prescribed by conventional medicine when something goes wrong. Ayurvedic medicine is just one facet of a complete Ayurvedic philosophy and way of life. It recognizes that most people can be characterized into various basic categories, and it offers dietary and exercise regimes suited to each of these. You can draw on the ancient principles of Ayurveda to help balance your energies by following a lifestyle suited to your particular character and body type. At the same time, recognizing the type of person you are will enhance your self awareness and help you to appreciate how your lifestyle is impinging and perhaps detracting from your current state of health and well-being. Ayurveda is the origin of many branches of complementary therapies today and uses colour infusions and herbal remedies, as well as crystal-healing, aromatherapy and massage, to help return the body to health. It truly is an all-round healing therapy that is very effective and appeals to a great many people.

All three natural therapies described here, herbalism, homeopathy and ayurveda, take time to examine the various symptoms of a person's illness and usually also offer preventative advice for the future. Perhaps it is this overall evaluation of the illness and then relating it to the whole person, combined with the self-help advice, that sets apart many complementary therapies from conventional medical practices. There is no doubt that it is refreshing to take back some of the responsibility for our own health, and

encouraging to know that we can work with our own bodies and with nature by using the materials they have to offer to keep us well. Although there are some uncontrollable external factors that affect our health, armed with a little knowledge of complementary medicine, we can enjoy vastly improved health, enabling us to live and enjoy our lives to the full.

# herbalism

herbalism herbalism

All over the world, people have used plants not only as food but also as medicines. Traditional knowledge of herbal remedies used to be passed from generation to generation, but nowadays this is rare.

Fortunately, the countryside still produces wonderful herbs and many can be grown in the garden. Getting to know the plants growing around you can be a relaxing pleasure in itself. If you learn about their various properties, you can use them to help you feel more healthy and better able to cope with everyday problems. Very simple remedies can easily be made from dried or fresh herbs, and substituting an excellent herb tea for stimulating drinks such as tea, coffee and cola will help you to relax and reduce your tension levels.

Herbs, like people, are complex and variable organic structures. Each plant contains many different constituents which together give a unique taste and range of actions. Particularly active constituents have been isolated and copied by pharmacists to produce medicines such as aspirin. However, using the whole plant has a much more subtle effect, and generates far fewer side effects. Herbalists therefore prefer to use the whole plant to treat the whole person. We are all unique and react to life in different ways; just as we all have special preferences for various foods, each of us responds best to particular herbs.

# the nervous system

It is easily overlooked, but the nervous system is like the key component in a highly complex computer. It regulates and fine tunes, analyses information and decides on the best course of action; it is an extremely sophisticated kind of mechanism. That is why looking after the nervous system is one of the most important things you can do. Here are some excellent ways of making sure that you relax and keep feeling well.

## The Effects of Stress

The involuntary or autonomic nervous system has two divisions. The sympathetic part prepares you for action and initiates the "fight or flight" response. The parasympathetic system is responsible for the body's "housekeeping", ensuring good digestion, assimilation of nutrients, detoxification and elimination of waste products. The sympathetic system allows you to respond to any stimulation, making the heart and lungs more active when necessary and suppressing natural processes such as digestion.

All life follows a natural rhythm, with periods of activity followed by periods of rest. This is as it should be. Too much stimulation, or an over-reaction to stimulation, leads to stress. If you are subjected to excess stimulation, sympathetic activities become dominant or habitual and may reach a state of exhaustion, reducing your ability to react and cope appropriately with new stresses. This can cause forgetfulness, panic, exhaustion or increased vulnerability to infection. At the same time, reduced parasympathetic activity can cause all sorts of digestive and nutritional debilities as well as poor elimination, which in turn can result in problems with the skin, muscles or joints.

*Lavender oil rubbed into the temples will encourage relaxation, and gradually ease a headache.*

## Helpful Herbs

The nervous system co-ordinates all the highly complex activities that manage to keep us functioning efficiently and well. They help us rapidly, unconsciously adjust to all kinds of constantly changing stimuli. The following pages clearly describe some of the highly valuable, beautiful plants growing right across the world which, among their many properties, help give back-up and support to the nervous system. Herbalists have named these very important plants, the nervines.

## Choosing the Right Remedies

Like all herbs, nervines have a wide range of actions. It is important that you choose the one that applies to your own symptoms of stress, and to which you feel naturally drawn. Knowing, growing, harvesting and drying herbs (which is quite easily done) will help you to appreciate them much more. You may well discover that a symptom that is particularly troubling can in fact be treated by several different remedies.

*Simply meandering down paths of richly scented lavender can quickly help to raise the spirits.*

### Nervous Tonics

These plants are used to aid recovery from stress and are particularly useful when we feel in any way debilitated and exhausted after an illness, prolonged pressure or even a trauma. They will improve the health and functioning of nervous tissue by invigorating and restoring it.

Some act as gentle stimulants while others are in fact slightly more sedating. Your choice will depend on whether nervous debility makes you hyperactive (in which case choose relaxing nervines) or restless, depressed and tired (in which case you must choose stimulating nervines).

### Stimulating Tonics:

- Mugwort (Artemisia vulgaris)
- Wild Oats (Avena sativa)
- St John's Wort (Hypericum perforatum)
- Sage (Salvia officinalis)
- Damiana (Turnera diffusa)

### Relaxing Tonics:

- Wood Betony (Stachys betonica)
- Skullcap (Scutellaria lateriflora)
- Vervain (Verbena officinalis)

### Stimulants

Some plants, such as coffee and tea, stimulate our nervous system without nourishing it. Since such over-stimulation is exhausting, additional herbal stimulants are rarely used. But there is a place for gently stimulating nervines. For example, Mugwort is beneficial during convalescence and Rosemary, by helping stimulate blood flow to the head, is used to tackle and reduce tension headaches.

- Rosemary (Rosmarinus officinalis)

### Relaxants and Sedatives

You can use relaxing nervines to calm yourself down and prevent over-stimulation. All these valuable herbs will help encourage rest and sleep. In any event some, like the Passion Flower and Lime Blossom, are excellent garden plants and help create a marvellous soothing atmosphere; a garden made for quietly walking round, inhaling the excellent scents, filled with a wide range of colours.

- Lady's Mantle (Alchemilla xanthochlora)
- Pasque Flower (Anemone pulsatilla)
- Chamomile (Chamaemelum nobile and Chamomilla recutita)
- Californian Poppy (Eschscholtzia californica)
- Hops (Humulus lupulus)
- Lavender (Lavandula spp.)
- Motherwort (Leonurus cardiaca)
- Lemon Balm (Melissa officinalis)
- Peppermint (Mentha piperita)
- Marjoram (Origanum vulgare)
- Passion Flower (Passiflora incarnata)
- Lime Blossom (Tilia x europaea)
- Cramp Bark (Viburnum opulus)
- Valerian (Valeriana officinalis)

### Adaptogens

- Siberian Ginseng (Eleutheroccocus senticosus)
- Korean Ginseng (Panax spp.)

### Other useful Herbs

- Borage (Borage officinalis)
- Licorice (Glycyrrhiza glabra)
- Evening Primrose (Oenothera biennis)
- Chaste Tree (Vitex agnus-castus)

## Taking Herbal Preparations

Like other medicines, herbal remedies must be taken at the appropriate time and in a suitable manner tailored to the individual. For example, in cases of pregnancy, no strong herbal teas should be taken during the first trimester, even if they would otherwise relieve stress because the body is in too sensitive a state. Likewise, young children, whose bodies are also very labile, should not take Peppermint or Sage tea, they may suffer an adverse reaction. It is commonsense to avoid ready-made herbal mixes that contain sugar, the sugar will only create an additional burden for the body, reducing its ability to cope. Where it is possible, the cause of the stress should be removed, and everything done to support the person at this time.

*Herbal teas are easily made in a wide range of flavours. They are a gentle and simple way to soothe both body and mind.*

# the herb garden

Herb gardens are easy to make and quickly stocked. Get a catalogue from a specialist seed supplier and you will probably find that they have eight or so different kinds of Basil from Europe and the Far East, with herbs like Coriander (cilantro) and Cumin. Growing them is incredibly easy. In most cases, pick regularly to encourage plenty of fresh, new tasty shoots. You will quickly see the benefits in the kitchen and your health.

## PLANTING HERBS

You do not need very much space to grow herbs: a small border, or even a collection of containers, will provide a perfectly good supply. But if you do have the room, a large herb garden offers the chance to try fun designs like a circle of triangular beds pointing in to a focal point such as a small statue or painted urn.

### Soil and Site

Most herbs are undemanding and quick to grow. They are essentially wild plants, and do not require rich, highly cultivated soil. Many of the most useful herbs, such as Sage, Thyme, Rosemary and Lavender, are natives of southern Europe and will not survive heavy clay soils or water-logged conditions. Many moisture-loving plants, such as Lemon Balm, Mint and Valerian, will grow happily in a light soil, though not in conditions of total drought. A sunny, sheltered position protected from strong biting winds will suit all the plants, though some, such as the more tender Lemon Verbena and Bay, will need protecting in bad winters.

### Design

A formal layout of small beds dissected by paths provides a satisfying framework for the lax, untidy growth of many herbs. It also makes sure that you can easily tend and pick when necessary. A single species to each bed can look highly effective, evoking the magical, atmospheric style of medieval herb gardens. In contrast, an informal cottage garden provides plenty of scope for imaginative, exuberant planting with herbs cleverly mixed in with flowers. Raised beds or a lively collection of attractive containers make easy-to-control, self-contained areas.

*A perfect example of a well-tended herb garden, with symmetrical beds and wide paths for easy access. The plants thrive in this warm, sheltered corner of the garden.*

# EXPERIENCING HERBS

Identifying, growing and harvesting herbs can be a marvellous, healing experience itself. Handling herbs brings you closer to nature and increases your appreciation of the vitality of plants.

## Growing

The quickest way to acquire herbs that will help you stay healthy is to grow them yourself. You can easily grow most from seed. This means that you will be sure what they are, and that they will have been grown safely and organically, without the use of any chemical sprays. Most of the herbs used in the remedies on the following pages will grow extremely well in temperate climates. In fact many are often regarded as weeds, and actually thrive on patches of spare ground despite getting no care and attention whatsoever.

*Many of the culinary herbs we use today were distributed throughout Europe by the Roman army.*

## Gathering

The aerial parts of herbs (the flowers, stems and leaves) should be gathered for use or for drying when the plants are in bud and totally dry. That means early morning when the sun has dried the dew. Roots should be dug in the autumn, cleaned and roughly chopped into very small pieces.

If you harvest from the wild, make quite sure that you have identified the plant correctly (use a good wild flower book) and that it has not been polluted by fertilizers, pesticides or car fumes. Never pick so much that you reduce next year's growth.

## Drying

Spread out your herbs on a rack to dry naturally in an airy position, out of direct sunlight. Alternatively, tie them in loose bundles and hang them from a beam, or dry them in an oven at a very low heat.

## Storing

Always make sure that you store dried herbs in airtight containers, kept well away from the light, and do not forget to label and date them. They will keep for up to six months, but the sooner they are used the better and fresher the flavour. (When they are kept for too long they look dull and taste of sawdust.) If you are in any way worried about over-drying your herbs, try storing them in a freezer instead. This is a particularly good technique for herbs such as Lemon Balm and Parsley, which quickly lose their flavour when they are dried.

## Buying

Many shops stock dried herbs. Buy these only if they seem fresh – they should be brightly coloured and strongly aromatic.

Some herbal remedies are now readily available over the counter in the form of capsules, tablets or tinctures. These are usually of good quality. Choose the simpler ones that tell you exactly the type and quantity of herb involved.

*Lime Blossom is abundant for easy picking in both the countryside and urban areas during early summer.*

# herbal preparations

Herbs are multi-talented. They can be used in the kitchen, fresh or dried, and to tackle a wide range of ailments from hyperactivity to insomnia. They even provide a refreshing tonic when you are feeling down-and-out. In fact, you can take herbal remedies internally as teas, decoctions and tinctures, or applied externally as soothing, relaxing oils and conditioners. Best of all, they guarantee gorgeous perfumes.

## MAKING TEAS

Herbal teas are also called infusions or tisanes. They are a simple and delicious way of extracting the goodness and flavour from the aerial parts of herbs. You can use either fresh or dried herbs to make such teas; note you need to use twice as much fresh plant material as dried. If you find the taste of some herb teas rather bitter, then try sweetening them with a little honey. Alternatively, try adding extra flavour by stirring the tea with a Licorice stick, or adding ginger.

**1** Put your herb(s) into a pot. Standard-strength tea is made with 1 tsp dried or 2 tsp fresh herbs to 1 cup of water.

**2** Strain and drink as required. Teas can be drunk cold as well as hot. Cold teas are thoroughly invigorating.

## MAKING DECOCTIONS

Infusing in boiling water is not enough to extract the constituents from roots or bark. This much tougher, harder, inflexible plant material needs to be broken up into far smaller pieces by chopping or crushing with a sharp knife.

Next, place every tiny scrap of this rough-cut material into a stainless steel, glass or enamelled pan, but absolutely not aluminium. Fill up with cold water, and gradually bring to the boil. Finally cover and simmer for about 15 minutes. The resulting liquid is what is called a decoction. Strain it and flavour, if necessary, and drink while it is still warm.

**1** Harvest root and bark in the colder months. Trim the aerial parts of the plant away from the root.

**2** Wash the roots thoroughly in cold water, ensuring they are perfectly clean, then chop into small pieces.

### Nervine Decoctions

- Cramp Bark
- Licorice
- Valerian

Avoid using Licorice if you suffer from high blood pressure.

**3** Fill a pan with cold water and add 1 tsp of the chopped herb per cup. Boil and simmer for 10–15 minutes.

**4** Strain and cool before drinking. Decoctions can be kept for 24 hours in the fridge. Drink reheated or cold.

## MAKING TINCTURES

Sometimes it is more convenient to take a spoonful of medicine than make a tea or decoction. Tinctures are made by steeping herbs in a mixture of alcohol and water. The alcohol extracts the medicinal constituents, and it also acts as an excellent preservative.

Herb syrups make good remedies for giving to children. They also improve the taste of herbs that might be bitter, such as Motherwort and Vervain.

**1** Place 100 g/3½ oz dried herbs or 300g/11 oz fresh herbs in a jar.

**2** Add 250ml/8fl oz/1 cup vodka and 250ml/8fl oz/1 cup water.

### Making Syrups

**1** Place 500g/1¼lb sugar/honey in a pan; add 1 litre/1¾ pints/4 cups water.
**2** Heat gently, stirring to dissolve,
**3** Add 150g/5oz plant material and heat gently for 5 minutes.
**4** Turn off the heat; steep overnight.
**5** Strain and store in an airtight container for future use. Since the sugar acts as a preservative, a herb syrup will keep for 18 months.

**3** Leave the herbs to steep in the liquid for a month, preferably on a sunny windowsill. Gently shake the jar daily.

**4** Strain and store the tincture in a dark glass bottle where it will keep well for approximately 18 months.

## COLD INFUSED OILS

Herbal oils are suitable for external use when having a massage, or as bath oils or hair and skin conditioners. Cold infused oils are quite simple to prepare. Macerate freshly cut herbs in vegetable oil for up to two weeks, but no more. Give the jar a daily shake. Finally drain off the oil, and squeeze the excess liquid out of the herbs. You will find that chamomile invariably gives excellent results.

**1** Fill a glass storage jar with the flowers or leaves of your chosen dried herb.

**2** Pour in a vegetable oil to cover the herbs; try sunflower or grape seed oil.

### Herb Oil Infusions

• Chamomile
• Lavender
• Marjoram
• Rosemary
• St John's Wort

Do not put St John's Wort oil on the skin before going into bright sunshine for fear of an adverse reaction.

**3** Stand the jar for two weeks on a windowsill to steep. Shake daily.

**4** Strain. For a stronger infusion, renew the herbs in the oil every two weeks.

herbal recipes

herbal recipes

# herbal recipes

In today's high-tech, high-speed world it is virtually impossible not to encounter stress, and stress at even alarmingly high levels. It can strike going to work when you get stuck in a gridlock traffic jam, at work with faxes, e-mails and meetings, and when you get back home and suddenly have to cope with meals and children. In fact, many people find that getting quality, quiet time for themselves is becoming increasingly difficult, if not impossible. But while you cannot always avoid stress, there are plenty of things you can do to help yourself cope better when life suddenly presents a barrage of testing, difficult challenges.

A good, healthy diet really does make a significant difference. It is therefore absolutely essential that you eat proper, healthy meals packed with vitamin-rich fruit and vegetables, and totally avoid artificial additives. If you miss these extra flavours, you will find that you get a far greater range using fresh or dried herbs, and of course they offer plenty of extra goodness.

Also, try as hard as you can to reduce your intake of such stimulants as tea, coffee, alcohol and cola. Instead, drink plenty of water and invigorating herbal teas. All kinds of flavours are becoming increasingly available. You simply choose what you like, and that can include Anise, Chamomile, Lemon Verbena, Lime Blossom, Mint, and Sage. They are all incredibly refreshing. Even better, you can grow these herbs in pots or in the garden, where you know they have been organically raised.

Exercise is equally important for all kinds of reasons. It dispels excess adrenaline and improves relaxation and sleep. Swimming prevents your joints from becoming stiff and gives the body a marvellous feeling of freedom. Exercise also tones up your muscles, keeps you in shape, and helps shed excess weight. In short, it keeps you feeling alert, well and able.

One of the biggest problems of stress is that it can all too easily disrupt your appetite and your ability to rest. In turn, such disruption makes you even less able to cope with any setbacks and problems. You get pulled into a depressing, downward spiral. One of the best ways to break out of this pattern is to use herbal remedies to improve your digestion, to help you relax, and to improve your adaptability.

The recipes that follow are designed to help you through difficult times. As long as you do not exceed the doses stated, and are sure that you are using the right plant, it is safe to experiment with these suggestions. But do seek professional help if a problem persists.

# key stress symptoms

While some degree of stress is an inevitable part of modern life, there are fortunately several significant ways of tackling it. They should help make sure that your day is not ruined by a tense neck or a nervous stomach. In fact some ways, such as using using excellent massage oils, are so incredibly relaxing, refreshing and enjoyable that they could well become part of your daily routine.

## CALMING ANXIETY

Everyone knows exactly what it feels like to be excited, but inappropriate or excessive excitement, often combined with frustration, creates anxiety. In this state, the body produces too much adrenaline. It is primed for "fight or flight" but neither is possible. The heart races, muscles tense and the chest expands. Anxiety can cause many symptoms, including palpitations, sweating, irritability and sleeplessness. In these situations, Rescue Remedy, which is bought ready-made, is useful.

*Two drops of Rescue Remedy on the tongue can help prevent a panic attack, and give you ease of mind.*

## RELAXING TENSE MUSCLES

Muscles can tense as a result of anxiety which often causes slightly raised shoulders or contracted back muscles. The effort of maintaining your muscles in this semi-contracted state is tiring, possibly causing spasms and bad postural habits. The neck stiffens and the back may ache. Tight neck muscles can also hinder blood flowing to the head, creating tension headaches. Moving frequently will release the muscles. Rotate your head or stand and stretch, and take breaks from working or driving. Gently massaging the neck with oil can help.

*Tension can build up in the neck and shoulders, causing stiffness.*

### Cold Infused Oil of Lavender

Fill a glass jar with lavender heads and cover with clear vegetable oil. Allow to steep on a windowsill, shaking the jar every day. Strain and bottle.

The oil can be used for massaging into a stiff neck or back. It can also be added to the bath to keep your skin soft and perfumed, while also encouraging relaxation.

Lavender is an extremely talented herb. It has traditionally been used as a sedative helping combat anxiety and tension. A few drops of infused oil added to your favourite massage oil will also help relax your over-tense muscles. Similar oils can be made from Marjoram (which is anti-spasmodic) and Rosemary.

### Herbal Remedies

To help your nervous system readjust and adapt, consider the value of:
- Skullcap
- St John's Wort
- Vervain
- Wild Oats
- Wood Betony

Choose whichever one suits you best and combine it with a specific remedy for the symptom that is causing you most problems.
- To ease palpitations: Motherwort or Passion Flower.
- To reduce sweating: Motherwort or Valerian.
- To help you sleep: Passion Flower.

*Chamomile tea makes an ideal after-dinner drink.*

## DIGESTIVES

Many people suffer from digestive upsets when they are stressed. This is because the "fight or flight" activity of the sympathetic nervous system tends to suppress digestive processes. The result may be indigestion, loss of appetite, wind, diarrhoea or even an irritable bowel.

The three recipes below have all been specially designed to help relax the nervous system, encouraging parasympathetic activity and reducing any signs of spasm in the gut.

### To Calm Butterflies

Nervous stomachs can be quickly settled by Chamomile, Hops and Lemon Balm combined in a tea, or simply select the best combination for you. Lemon Balm and Chamomile can be taken as frequently as you like.

Put 1 tsp each Lemon Balm, dried Chamomile flowers and Peppermint into a small tea pot or cafetière. Fill with boiling water and allow to steep for at least 10 minutes. Strain and drink at least three times a day or after meals.

| **Herbal Remedies** | |
| --- | --- |
| • Chamomile | • Hops |
| • Cramp Bark | • Lemon Balm |
| • Cumin | • Licorice |
| • Fennel, Caraway, Dill | • Peppermint |

### To Relieve Wind and Colic

In a small saucepan, boil 1 tsp each Fennel seeds and Cramp Bark with about 300ml/½ pint/1¼ cups water. Add 1 tsp dried Peppermint. Allow to steep for 10 minutes. Strain and drink.

### To Ease Constipation

Make a decoction of Cramp Bark and Fennel as above, but add 1 tsp Licorice root. If the constipation is proving to be an unpleasant, recurrent condition, 1 tsp Linseeds added daily to your breakfast cereal can be very helpful.

The same amount can also be soaked in hot water for about two hours, and drunk before going to bed and again, if necessary, early the next morning when you wake. If the problem is not eased or solved then it is important that you consult your doctor at the first opportunity. Generally, the best way to avoid an attack of constipation is to make sure that you are regularly having a balanced, healthy diet which includes plenty of fresh fruit, vegetables and roughage on a daily basis.

### Contraindications

Some herbs should only be used at certain times and not if you are suffering certain other symptoms. For example, since Hops are a sedative, they should only be taken at night, and are not suitable if you are depressed or lacking in sexual energy. Likewise, Licorice should be avoided if you have high blood pressure or oedema. Always consult a medical doctor if in any doubt.

# revitalizing recipes

You do not have to be so ill that you are completely confined to bed to take some of the excellent revitalizing herbal remedies now available. Many are purpose designed as a refreshing pick-me-up or tonic to get you through testing emotional and physical times – the bad, dark days – when the mind and body might otherwise become tired and sluggish. Such recipes are nature's way of keeping you healthy.

## NERVOUS EXHAUSTION

It is much more likely that you will get ill or depressed after or during a long period of hard work, or from a whole battery of emotional demands. This can easily happen to teachers, for example, at the end of term, or to those who have to care for disabled or sick relations on a long-term basis. You will find that herbal remedies help to give your nervous system plenty of vital support at such testing, difficult times. To make a revitalizing tea, mix equal portions of all the dried herbs listed. Put 3–4 tsp of the mixture into a pot with a lid. Add 600ml/1 pint/2½ cups boiling water. Steep for 10 minutes, strain, and drink 3–4 cups a day.

### Herbal Remedies

- Borage
- Licorice
- Skullcap
- St John's Wort
- Wild Oats
- Wood Betony

*Make a relaxing herbal tea from a blend of supportive herbs whenever you are feeling exhausted and too tired to cope.*

*Borage, like Licorice, restores the adrenal glands.*

## TONICS FOR CONVALESCENCE

Remember that even if your symptoms have gone, your body needs time to recover after an illness. A tonic is extremely useful. Wild Oats and St John's Wort support the nervous system, Vervain promotes relaxation and digestion, and Licorice restores the adrenal glands. Vitamin C supplements should be continued for several weeks after an illness. Alfalfa sprouts are also high in vitamins and minerals. Also note that rest is very important.

### Tonic Tea

Put ½ tsp of each of one of the dried herbs listed below into a small pot. Add boiling water. Flavour with Peppermint to taste. (Avoid Licorice if you suffer from high blood pressure or oedema.) Allow to steep for 10 minutes. Strain. Drink three or four cups, warm, each day for at least three weeks.

### Herbal Remedies

- Borage
- Licorice
- St John's Wort
- Vervain
- Wild Oats

*St John's Wort thrives in a bright, open sunny position.*

## RELIEVING WINTER BLUES

The old herbalists thought that the appearance of a plant held a clue to its healing action. For instance, Pilewort (Lesser Celandine) has roots that resemble haemorrhoids, and it does indeed make an effective ointment for piles. The flowers of St John's Wort resemble nothing so much as the sun. The plant thrives in sunlight and is known to have anti-depressant effects. There is no better herb than this to take if you are depressed in the winter, when sunlight is in short supply.

Wild Oats also help by strengthening the nervous system and keeping you warm. Rosemary, an evergreen plant, will improve circulation to the head and keep the mind clear. Also, Ginseng capsules can be taken for a month in the early autumn to help you adapt to the difficult transition between seasons.

### Winter Brightener

Combine 2 tsp dried St John's Wort with 1 tsp dried Rosemary. Add 250ml/8fl oz/1 cup boiling water. Allow to steep for 10 minutes and then strain. One cup alone is not enough. Drink three times a day throughout the winter.

| Herbal Remedies | |
| --- | --- |
| • Ginseng | • St John's Wort |
| • Rosemary | • Wild Oats |

## LIFTING DEPRESSION

Depression is a very good illustration of the close connection that exists between the body and mind: physical and emotional energy are both depleted when you are in a depressed state. Both will benefit from a healthy diet that includes plenty of raw, vital foods, nuts, seeds and B vitamins. A multi-vitamin and mineral supplement is an effective kick-start that will give you an excellent lift. But do not undermine its effect by indulging in stimulants, such as caffeine, because they tend to exhaust both the body and mind.

The refreshing, restorative tea described below is a marvellous, tasty way of restoring the health of your nervous system. It has a slight, barely noticeable, stimulating effect.

### Restorative Tea

Mix equal parts of each of the dried herbs listed in the box below. Put 2 tsp of the mixture into a pot. Add 600ml/1 pint/2½ cups boiling water. Allow to steep for 10 minutes and then strain. Drink one cup of this excellent tea three times a day.

| Herbal Remedies | |
| --- | --- |
| • Damiana | • Wild Oats |
| • St John's Wort | |

*There are many tasty ways of incorporating the goodness of Oats in your diet, including home-made snacks such as biscuits.*

# headache and night-time remedies

From time to time everyone suffers from headaches and bad sleepless nights. Occasional attacks are just about bearable, but when they become a regular feature and interrupt your life, especially your sex life, it is clearly time to act. All these herbal solutions, ranging from baths and teas to massages, have one aim: to give you back your healthy life as quickly as possible.

## RELIEVING TENSION HEADACHES

Headaches are a common symptom of stress. Often they are caused by tension in the neck and upper back muscles. This can prevent adequate blood supply to the head and thus lead to pain. Both massage and exercise can ease this kind of headache.

### Scented Baths

Pour a few drops of essential oil or infused oil into a hot bath, lie back and relax. Better, tie a bunch of herbs under the hot tap as you fill the bath. Rub two drops of essential oil of Lavender mixed with 1 tsp water on the head when stressed.

### Soothing Tea

Put 1 tsp dried Wood Betony and ½ tsp dried Lavender or Rosemary into a cup. Top up with boiling water and leave for 10 minutes, before straining and drinking. Repeat hourly.

| Herbal remedies | |
|---|---|
| • Lavender | • Rosemary |

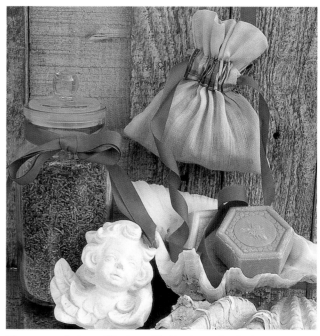

*Hang a muslin bag of fresh or dried herbs under the hot tap.*

*Help yourself beat a hangover by taking a herbal remedy.*

## HANGOVER REMEDIES

Most people know what a hangover feels like – a combination of headache, nausea, fuzzy head and depression. Most of these symptoms are connected with the liver being overloaded. Bitter herbs stimulate the liver and speed up its ability to detoxify. Vervain is bitter and Lavender aids digestion; both herbs also lift the spirits. If you have a hangover it is also advisable to drink plenty of water and take extra vitamin C.

### Morning-After Tea

Put 1 tsp dried Vervain and ½ tsp Lavender flowers into a pot. Add 600ml/1 pint/2½ cups boiling water and cover to keep in the volatile oils. Steep for 10 minutes. Strain and sweeten with a little honey. Sip through the day until you start to feel better.

| Herbal Remedies | |
|---|---|
| • Lavender | • Vervain |

## REVITALIZING THE LIBIDO

Depression or anxiety can all too easily hinder and interrupt your sex life. This may be because your energy is too low, or it may in fact be connected with a hormone imbalance. Damiana stimulates both the nervous and hormonal systems, and it has vital constituents which convert to hormones in the body. Vervain is good at releasing tension and stress, and it was traditionally used as an aphrodisiac. Wild Oats and Ginger root are both considered stimulating too.

### Energizing Tea

Put 1 tsp dried Damiana and 1 tsp dried Vervain into a pot. Add 600ml/1 pint/2½ cups of boiling water. Leave to steep for 10 minutes. Strain and flavour with Licorice, Ginger or honey, as you prefer. Drink two cups a day.

| **Herbal Remedies** | |
|---|---|
| • Damiana | • Vervain |
| • Ginger | • Wild Oats |

*Teas or decoctions made with the right herbs can help restore energy of all kinds, including sexual energy.*

## ENHANCING SLEEP

There are many different types of insomnia, and the causes are varied. If you really cannot sleep then it is best to experiment with the remedies below to find the one herb or combination of herbs that suits you best. If the problem is long term and you have not been sleeping well for a period of time, then take a nervous system tonic to improve your well being.

In the evenings, drink teas that have been made from relaxing herbs. Lavender oil in a hot bath before bed and on the pillow will also help. You could even try using a Hop pillow. Furthermore, it is important to give yourself plenty of time at the end of the day to relax and wind down. Exercise, meditation and yoga are all good at helping you fall asleep.

*You can make or buy a herb pillow to encourage sound sleep.*

### Sleepy Tea

Put 1 tsp each dried Chamomile, Vervain and Lemon Balm into a pot. Add about 600ml/1 pint/2½ cups boiling water. Leave to steep for 10 minutes. Strain and drink one cup after supper. Warm the rest and drink before going to bed.

If you continue to have problems sleeping, add a decoction of 1 tsp Valerian root or ½ tsp dried Hops or Californian Poppy to this blend of herbs.

| **Herbal Remedies** | |
|---|---|
| • Californian Poppy | • Passion Flower |
| • Chamomile | • Valerian |
| • Hops | • Vervain |
| • Lemon Balm | |

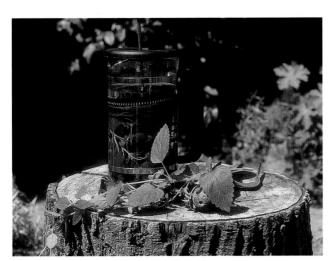

*Chamomile tea is not only beneficial but extremely refreshing.*

# herbal facials
The skin is all too sensitive to poor health and is easily damaged, not in dramatic ways but in gradual, subtle ways that can easily make it dry or even quite inflamed. Many people think that such damage is an inevitable part of living and ageing, and that there is nothing you can do about it, but fortunately they are wrong. There are plenty of steps you can take to keep your skin looking healthy and beautiful.

## PREPARING THE SKIN

A facial steam treatment is an excellent way of deep-cleaning the skin. Always close the pores afterwards with a skin toner, or a face mask. Keep your face about 30cm/12in above the bowl, and cover your head and the bowl with a towel for a few minutes. Steam facials should be avoided by people with thread veins.

Pore cleansers can be useful if you suffer from acne. Combine a weekly Marigold facial with a diet full of fresh, raw salad vegetables and avoid refined starches. This, combined with plenty of exercise, will relieve the skin of some of the cleansing activity (the acne) being carried out by the skin.

### Steam Cleanser for Normal Skin

Put 40g/1½oz fresh or 15g/½oz dried Chamomile flowers into a bowl with 600ml/1 pint/2½ cups boiling water. Leave to stand for 30 minutes, and then strain. In a pan, re-heat the infusion and pour into a bowl. Use as directed above.

### Pore Cleansers for Problem Skin

Follow the steps above, but use Marigold petals instead. Also add 5ml/1 tsp of distilled Witch Hazel to the infusion.

*A steam treatment relaxes and softens the skin. Make it with an infusion of dried herbs, or simply float fresh herbs in boiling water.*

*Wheatgerm oil, honey and egg yolk are all nourishing for dry skin.*

## FACE MASKS

Herbal face masks tighten the skin, leaving it feeling smooth and fresh. Do not use them too often as they can be over-stimulating. Comfrey and Rosewater masks are excellent for dry skin, whereas Parsley and Sage masks will help oily skin. Apply the mask mixture evenly to the face, but avoid the areas around the eyes. Leave for 10–15 minutes, and then rinse off with water.

### Soothing Mask for Dry Skin

Place 6 Comfrey leaves in 150ml/¼ pint/⅔ cup boiling water, stir, cool and strain. Mix 15ml/1 tbsp of this infusion with 30ml/2 tbsp ground Wild Oats, 1 egg yolk, 5ml/1 tsp honey, 5ml/1 tsp Rosewater, 5 drops wheatgerm oil, and a little milk to mix.

### Purifying Mask for Oily Skin

Infuse 15g/½oz fresh Parsley, 15g/½oz fresh Sage in 300ml/½ pint/1¼ cups boiling water. Mix 30–45ml/2–3 tbsp of this with 30ml/2 tbsp ground Wild Oats, 15ml/1 tbsp fuller's earth, 1 egg white, and 5ml/1 tsp Lemon juice.

## CLEANSERS AND SCRUBS

Facial scrubs enliven the skin and encourage its self-cleansing activities. The gentle grains slough away the dead skin, stimulate the circulation and leave it looking revitalized and fresh. Scrubs are useful at any time of the year, but especially in the dark, cold winter months when skin lacks that healthy glow. They can be used in place of toner, but should be used before moisturizing the skin. Any perfumed petals, citrus skin or essential oils can be substituted into the recipes below.

To use, store the scrub in an airtight jar until it is required. When needed, mix to a soft paste with almond oil and using small circular movements, gently rub it into the skin. Rinse off with warm water and pat your face dry.

### Perfumed Petal Face Scrub

Mix together 45ml/3 tbsp skinned ground almonds, 45ml/3 tbsp medium oatmeal and 45ml/3 tbsp powdered milk. Use a coffee grinder to powder 30ml/2 tbsp dried Rose petals and add them to the mixture.

### Stimulating Citrus Scrub

Mix together 45ml/3 tbsp of each of the following: ground sunflower seeds, medium oatmeal, flaked sea salt and finely grated Orange peel, combine with 3 drops of grapefruit essential oil.

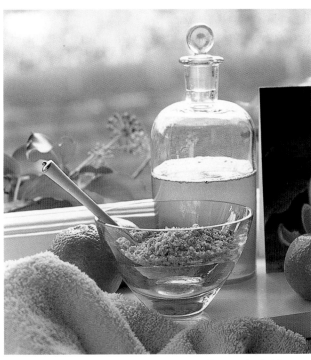

*Facial scrubs are very simple to make and of all the herbal beauty treatments they keep the longest.*

*Dark red Roses are best for colour. The toner on the left is made from fragrant 'Ena Harkness', with Elderflower on the right.*

## SKIN TONERS

Different formulations of skin tonics are used to soothe or stimulate the skin. Fine dry skin needs soothing with delicate herbal infusions or flower waters, while large-pored or oily skins can benefit from a stimulating tonic containing witch hazel.

### Orangeflower Toner for Normal Skin

Mix together 75ml/5 tbsp Orangeflower water with 25ml/1½ tbsp Rosewater. Store in a glass bottle.

### Rose Petal Toner for Sensitive Skin

Place 40g/1½oz fresh Rose petals, 600ml/1 pint/2½ cups boiling water and 15ml/1 tbsp cider vinegar in a bowl. Cover and leave to stand for approximately 2 hours. Strain the toner into a clean glass bottle.

### Lime Flower Toner for Mature Skin

Place 20g/¾oz fresh Lime flowers in a bowl with 90ml/6 tbsp boiling water. Leave to stand for about 2 hours then strain into a bottle. Add 10ml/2 tsp Rosewater into the bottle, shake gently and cover. This infusion will keep for 2–3 days if kept cool.

### Lavender Toner for Oily Skin

Combine 20g/¾oz fresh Lavender flowers with 90ml/6 tbsp boiling water and leave to stand for about 2 hours. Strain with a sieve or through a cloth. Add 25ml/1½ tbsp Witch Hazel to the mixture, stir and decant into a bottle.

# natural skin care
Your skin is the first and the most important protection you have against the outside world. If it is seen as an organ, then it is one of the body's main cleansing organs, and the one with the largest surface area. That is why it makes good sense to take excellent care of it. The simple moisturizing treatments described here will help preserve and enhance the beauty and function of your skin, keeping it in the best of health.

## MOISTURIZERS
Herbal moisturizing lotions are very easy to make and require only basic kitchen tools. The herbs recommended here are a good complement to the main moisturizing ingredients, but the oils, milk, cocoa butter and beeswax are the moisturizers while the herbs add more subtle properties to the creams and lotions.

### Bath Oil
Place 6 sprigs of Rosemary with vegetable oil in a jar and leave for 2 weeks, then strain. Beat together 2 eggs and 45ml/3 tbsp of Rosemary oil, then mix in 10ml/2 tbsp honey, 10ml/2 tsp baby shampoo, 15ml/1 tbsp vodka and 150ml/¼ pint/⅔ cup milk. Add 45ml/3 tbsp to the bath, and use the rest within a few days. Lemon Balm or Lavender can be substituted for the Rosemary.

### Body Lotion for Dry Skin
Melt 50g/2 oz coconut oil in a heatproof bowl placed over a pan of simmering water. Stir in 60ml/4 tbsp sunflower and 10ml/2tsp wheatgerm oils. Leave to cool, then add 10 drops of Orangeflower essence and pour into a jar to solidify.

*A marvellous bath lotion, made with honey and Rosemary oil, which will soon leave the skin looking healthy, smooth and silky.*

*Solid moisturizers, such as this Barrier Cream, can make lovely gifts if packaged imaginatively and then wrapped in cellophane.*

### Instant Moisturizer
Combine 300ml/½ pint/1¼ cups almond oil with 4 drops of Rose oil, or other perfumed oil. Keep in a small bottle and use by tipping the bottle neck against the skin.

### Moisturizer for Blemishes
Put 20g/¾ oz cocoa butter, 20ml/4 tsp beeswax granules and 75ml/5 tbsp almond oil in a bowl and melt over a pan of simmering water. In a separate pan, stir 10ml/2tsp borax in 175ml/6fl oz/¾ cup of Lavender water. When it has dissolved, add it to the beeswax mixture and stir to combine. Add 8 drops of Lavender essential oil, mix well and transfer to glass jars.

### Barrier Cream
Grate 75g/3oz unscented soap into a bowl, pour over 90ml/6 tbsp boiling water and stir until smooth. Combine 115g/4oz beeswax, 45ml/3 tbsp glycerine, 150ml/¼ pint/⅔ cup almond oil with 45ml/3 tbsp Orangeflower water and melt in a double boiler. Remove from the heat and whisk in the soap until it thickens. Stir in 25 drops of Citrus oil and pour into containers.

## HAND TREATMENTS

Gardening, winter weather, the daily grind of domestic chores and the demands of everyday living can all too easily take their toll on your hands. They can quickly become rough and sore, and even quite leathery, and the more quickly you tackle the problem the quicker your skin will become soft and supple again. This is particularly important if you like giving your partner a gentle massage. Use Roses to redress the balance.

### Rose Infusion

Put a handful of fragrant Rose petals into a bowl with 600ml/ 1 pint/2½ cups boiling water. Leave for 30 minutes, pour in 30ml/2 tbsp vodka, then strain.

### Rose Hand Mask

Put 45ml/3 tbsp medium or fine oatmeal, 30ml/2 tbsp Rose Infusion or triple-distilled Rosewater, 5ml/1 tsp almond oil, 5ml/ 1 tsp lemon juice and 5ml/1 tsp glycerine into a bowl and mix into a paste. Spread it on the backs of your hands and fingers and leave for 15 minutes, then rinse off with water and apply the Rose Hand Lotion.

### Rose Hand Lotion

Mix together 90ml/6 tbsp glycerine, 30ml/2 tbsp Rose Infusion and 10ml/2 tsp triple-distilled Rosewater. Add 10ml/2 tsp corn-flour (cornstarch) and beat until incorporated into the liquid.

*A lotion of Rosewater and glycerine keeps hands smooth.*

*Treat inflamed skin by gently applying soothing Marigold milk to the face, dabbing it on with cotton wool balls.*

## TREATMENTS FOR PROBLEM SKIN

The skin can suffer from numerous complaints, from cuts and scratches to life-long eczema. Herbalism has something to offer in each case, although the latter complaint may need professional help. When using these creams, test for sensitivity by applying a little of the cream to the wrist and leaving overnight. Keep all creams in clean jars or bottles in the refrigerator.

### Healing Ointment for Cuts and Scratches

Pack Marigold flowers into an airtight glass jar and leave on a sunny windowsill for 10 days. Strain off the oily liquid. Melt 90ml/6 tbsp petroleum jelly, 2.5ml/½ tsp paraffin wax and 1.5ml/¼ tsp lanolin in a double boiler. Add 10 drops of the marigold oil and mix.

### Soothing Ointment for Eczema

Infuse 25g/1oz dried Comfrey, Marigold or Evening Primrose with 475ml/16fl oz/2 cups boiling water, leave for 10 minutes, then strain. In a double boiler, melt 25g/1oz beeswax with 120ml/ 4fl oz/½ cup vegetable oil, remove from the heat and whisk in 25ml/1½ tbsp of the infusion drop by drop.

### Drying Tincture for Cold Sores

Place 100g/4oz dried Marigold petals with 250ml/8fl oz/1 cup vodka (30% alcohol or 60% proof). Leave for a month on a sunny windowsill. Gently shake the jar each day, then strain and store.

# hair treatments
Hair is all too often taken for granted, but it too needs sensitive care and attention, particularly against the ravages of city life, with smoke and heavy pollution, and even against the worst the elements can throw at it. Store-bought shampoos can be effective, but they do lack the personal touch. You can easily achieve this by making a simple herbal treatment, which will add a wonderful attractive shine and a marvellous instant scent.

## HERBAL SHAMPOOS
Much damage is caused to hair by washing it too frequently and by the detergents that it contains. This upsets the natural balance of oils and chemicals in the scalp and can create problems such as dandruff. Try these gentle shampoos instead.

### Soapwort Shampoo
Break up and chop 25g/1oz fresh Soapwort root, leaves and stem or 15g/½ oz dried Soapwort root and put it into a pan. Add 750ml/1¼ pints/3 cups plain water. Simmer for 20 minutes, then strain the herbs and add a dash of Lavender water or Eau-de-Cologne. Use as ordinary shampoo.

### Chamomile Shampoo
Infuse 25g/1 oz dried Chamomile flowers with 1 litre/1¾ pints/4 cups boiling water for 1 hour and then strain. Just before using mix 15ml/1 tbsp of the infusion with 60ml/4 tbsp Soapwort Shampoo and 5 drops Neroli essential oil.

*The effective cleansing properties of Soapwort (Saponaria officinalis) are due to the saponins which it contains.*

*Chamomile can be used for a lightening rinse. For extra effect also add it to your shampoo.*

## HERBAL HAIR RINSES
For keeping the hair shiny and to enhance its natural colour, try using the following rinses after shampooing. Simply stand over a bowl and pour through the hair and re-apply at least 6 times.

### Chamomile Rinse for Fair Hair
Infuse 25g/1oz dried Chamomile in 1 litre/1¾ pints/4 cups boiling water. in a large bowl for 1 hour, and then strain.

### Rosemary Rinse for Dark Hair
Infuse 40g/1½ oz fresh Rosemary in 1 litre/1¾ pints/4 cups boiling water in a bowl for 1 hour and then strain.

### Nettle Rinse for Dandruff
Infuse 25g/1oz fresh Nettle leaves in 1 litre/1¾ pints/4 cups boiling water overnight then strain. Add 30ml/2 tbsp cider vinegar and 30ml/2 tbsp Witch Hazel.

| Herbal Remedies | |
|---|---|
| • Chamomile | • Rosemary |

# caring for the mouth

Commercial mouth treatments are often harsh and contain chemicals that can affect the self-balancing and self-healing abilities of the mouth. Toothpastes may also contain detergents which can adversely affect the lining of the gut, and this can also cause problems. If you have time it is worth making your own tooth powders and mouthwashes, which can be adapted, when needed, to treat any upsets in the mouth.

## ORAL HYGIENE

The mouth is often one of the first places that tells us when we are run down. The most common symptom of this is mouth ulcers, and oral thrush is also quite common. The first priority to aid prevention and recovery is to eat plenty of fresh vegetables, raw and cooked, and have enough exercise and plenty of rest. Secondly, use a simple tooth powder or paste that will not interfere with the natural balance of good bacteria in the mouth that help to fight simple infections.

## Tooth Powder

Bake 25g/1oz fresh shredded Sage or Mint leaves with 60ml/4 tbsp sea salt or orris root at a very low temperature in the oven for 1 hour. Pound the mixture to a fine powder and use on a damp toothbrush. Note that if you are pregnant or planning a pregnancy, Sage should be avoided.

## Tooth Cleaners

Simpler herbal tooth cleaners include fresh Sage leaves rubbed over the teeth or Lemon peel can be rubbed over teeth to remove stains.

*A combination of shredded Sage leaves mixed with sea salt, baked and then powered, is traditionally used for cleaning teeth.*

*Chewing various seeds and spices to freshen and sweeten the breath is a widespread custom in the Far East.*

## BREATH FRESHENERS

Bad breath or halitosis is often symptomatic of a digestive problem or the onset of a cold and therefore may require the help of a professional herbalist or doctor. At other times, it is simply the result of eating too much garlic or spicy food. Whichever it is, this recipe will sweeten your breath.

## Refreshing Mouthwash

Simmer 5ml/1 tsp each of ground nutmeg, ground cloves, cardamom pods, caraway seeds and 15g/½oz dried Lemon Balm with 600ml/1 pint/2½ cups purified water. Strain and add 30ml/2 tbsp sweet sherry. Store in a clean bottle. Dilute 15–30ml/1–2 tbsp in a glass of water.

## Breath Enhancers

The following fresh herbs and dried spices can be chewed to freshen breath: Parsley, Watercress, Mint, seeds of Fennel, Star Anise, Cinnamon stick or cloves. Alternatively rinse your mouth with diluted rosewater.

# guide to herbs and their uses It has long been

known that herbs are an essential part of the kitchen, adding all kinds of flavours, and for

helping to relieve and cure a range of problems from migraines to wind (gas). The early physic

gardens in monasteries were really basic pharmacies stocking many of these essential plants. Do

not try and compete. Just grow those herbs that you know will help you feel much better.

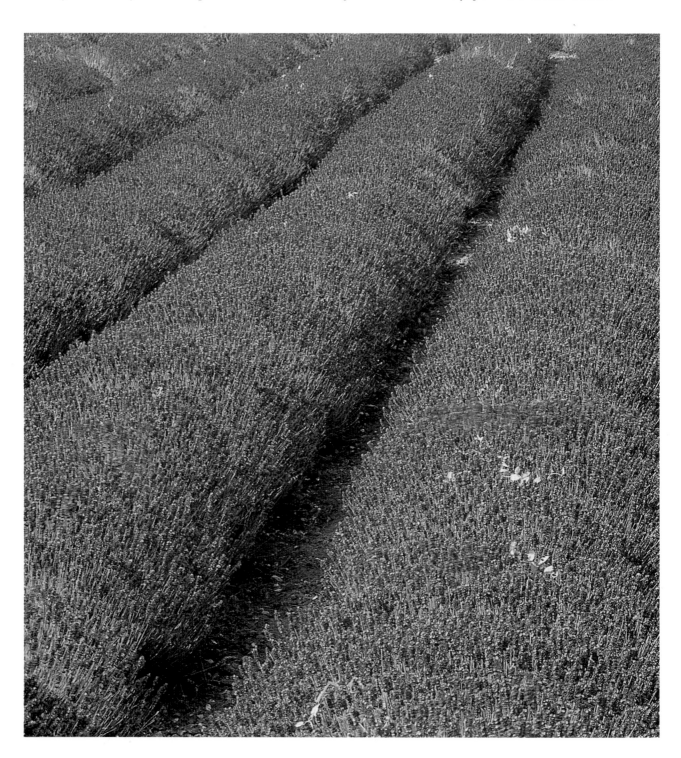

## USING HERBS

The herbs described on the following pages are a particularly useful group for helping tackle stress and various other common conditions. Reading the notes and studying the pictures will help you decide which would be most beneficial for you and your garden. After all, they should also help make a special relaxing feature. If planting them in groups, remember to put the tallest in the centre and the smaller ones around.

You may well want to try several as remedies before deciding which you find most helpful. Note that herbs do not usually work instantly, so do not be impatient and give them at least two weeks to take effect. If you do not feel better in three weeks, seek the help of a qualified practitioner. Herbs can also be used in various combinations, and you will find suggestions for putting them together to give additional benefits.

Since most of us would benefit from a nerve tonic during stressful times, choose the herbal remedy best suited to you.

For example, if when stressed you start to feel depressed, then look for a stimulating herbal tonic such as Wild Oats. If, however, stress makes you feel anxious and you start developing symptoms such as palpitations, sweating and sleeplessness, then turn to those herbs that have a relaxing effect.

Rescue Remedy, because it is not strictly herbal, but a Bach Flower remedy is not included in this directory, but it is readily available over the counter.

It is quite clear that some herbs are multi-talented. Borage gives a marvellous show of flowers and adds to the cottage garden, attracting plenty of bees. The leaves add a cucumber flavour to drinks, the flowers can garnish salads, and the oil lowers blood pressure. Lavender is another all-purpose herb, essential for pot-pourris and for a range of soothing treatments. If you find some plants do not succeed in certain parts of the garden, move them around until you find a more suitables place and you may well find that they perk up.

## LADY'S MANTLE

Alchemilla xanthochlora syn.
A. vulgaris, Virgin's Cape

The unusual leaves of this plant resemble a cloak, hence its common names. The name Alchemilla derives from the Arabic word for alchemy, signifying its power to help make a change. A larger species, Alchemilla mollis, is grown as a foliage plant. Lady's Mantle is a women's herb and helps balance menstrual cycles. As a douche or wash, an infusion helps sooth any itching or inflammation.

**n o t e s** • Parts used: Leaves and flowers.
• Dose: 1 tsp dried/2 tsp fresh to a cup of boiling water three times a day.

## PASQUE FLOWER

Anemone pulsatilla, Wind Flower

One of the most beautiful medicinal herbs with purple spring flowers. The common name comes from *Pasch* meaning Easter. Pasque Flower is a sedative, bactericidal, anti-spasmodic painkiller used to treat the reproductive organs. It is used against all types of pain affecting male and female genital organs.

**n o t e s** • Parts used: Dried leaves and flowers.
• Dose: A very low dose is needed – it is advisable to consult a herbalist.
**c a u t i o n :** Do not use the fresh plant.

## MUGWORT

Artemisia vulgaris

The "mother of herbs" grows robustly along roadsides and is said to protect the traveller. It is best described as a tonic with particular application to the digestive and nervous systems; it reduces nervous indigestion, nausea and irritability. As a womb tonic it helps regulate the menstrual cycle, reduces any associated period pain and PMS. It is also used to repel insects, including moths.

**n o t e s** • Parts used: Flowers and leaves.
• Dose: ¼–½ tsp three times a day.
**c a u t i o n :** Avoid in pregnancy.

## WILD OATS

Avena sativa

Oats are an excellent tonic to the nervous system. They slightly stimulate and are a long-term remedy for nervous exhaustion. They also help cope with shingles and herpes. Oats contain vitamin E, iron, zinc, manganese and protein and help reduce cholesterol.

**n o t e s** • Parts used: Seeds and stalks.
• Dose: There are many ways to take oats – in gruel, porridge, flapjacks, oatcakes and other dishes, as well as tea.
**c a u t i o n :** Oats are not always suitable for those who are sensitive to gluten.

## BORAGE
Borago officinalis

A strapping plant with lovely, luminous blue flowers. They make an attractive garnish to ice cream and cold summer puddings. Borage boosts the production of adrenaline and is useful in times of stress. It is also very nutritious, and helps to treat skin diseases and rheumatism.

**n o t e s** • Parts used: The leaves, flowers and seeds. The leaves need to be dried quite quickly and are best heated very gently in a cool oven until they are crisp.
• Dose: 1 tsp dried/2 tsp fresh to one cup of boiling water.

## CHAMOMILE
Chamomilla recutita or
Chamaemelum nobile

This pretty daisy is one of the better known herbs, possibly because it is so useful. Use the flowerheads alone in a tea or tincture to relax both the digestive function and those gut feelings that may sometimes disturb you. It makes a very suitable tea to drink late in the day because it has quite the opposite effect to that of coffee, which actually exacerbates tension and anxiety.

**n o t e s** • Parts used: Flower heads.
• Dose: 1 tsp dried/2 tsp fresh to a cup of boiling water.

## CALIFORNIAN POPPY
Eschscholzia californica

The beautiful, delicate flowers last for one day and are then replaced by long pointed seed pods. The stunning hot orange, yellow and pinkish colours of the blooms might account for its French name, *globe de soleil*. Californian Poppy is a gentle painkiller and sedative which reduces spasms and over-excitability.

**n o t e s** • Parts used: The whole plant
• Dose: 1 tsp dried herb to a cup of boiling water.
**c a u t i o n :** It is important to avoid this herb if you suffer from glaucoma.

## LICORICE
Glycyrrhiza glabra

A highly useful herb which has been cultivated since the Middle Ages for its sweet, aromatic roots. It aids digestion and reduces inflammation along the gut, loosening the bowels. Licorice heated in honey makes a soothing syrup, helping to soothe attacks of bronchitis and asthma.

**n o t e s** • Parts used: The root (Licorice sticks) or solidified juice in the form of black bars.
• Dose: 1 tsp to a cup of boiling water.
**c a u t i o n :** Not recommended for those with high blood pressure or oedema.

## HOP
Humulus lupulus

The name Hop comes from the Anglo-Saxon *hoppen*, "to climb": the twining fibrous stems may top 4.5m/15ft. Hops are taken as a bitter tonic helping both to improve digestion and to reduce any restlessness. It also has a sedative effect and will provoke deep sleep. The action is partly due to its volatile oils.

**n o t e s** • Parts used: Dried flowers from the female plant, called "strobiles".
• Dose: Not more than 1 tsp a day.
**c a u t i o n :** Avoid the use of Hops during any depressive illness.

## ST JOHN'S WORT
Hypericum perforatum

To be sure that you have the right plant, hold a leaf to the sun; the oil glands look like little holes. The plant is now well known for its anti-depressant action. It is a nerve tonic which helps nervous exhaustion and damage to nerves caused by diseases such as shingles.

**n o t e s** • Parts used: Flowering tops.
• Dose: 1 tsp dried/2 tsp fresh to a cup of boiling water, three times a day.
**c a u t i o n :** This remedy is best avoided when you are spending any time out in the garden when there is bright sunlight.

## GINSENG
Korean Ginseng, *Panax spp.*

By improving the production of adrenal hormones, Korean Ginseng helps the body to adapt to stress and resist disease. It should only be taken for short periods though. It benefits ME sufferers.

**n o t e s** • Parts used: Dried root.
• Dose: 1g per day.
**c a u t i o n :** Avoid the use of Ginseng during pregnancy or when taking other stimulants. Do not take high doses for more than six weeks without seeking expert advice. Stop taking Ginseng if it makes you feel agitated or if you develop a headache.

## LAVENDER
Lavandula spp.

Everybody knows this fragrant plant. Herbalists call it a thymoleptic, which means it raises the spirits. This, combined with its anti-infective action and relaxing properties, makes Lavender a powerful remedy. The essential oil is used externally for relaxation and to heal sores and burns. Lavender can also be taken internally in a tea or tincture. It is also an ideal remedy for irritation, indigestion and for the onset of a migraine attack.

**n o t e s** • Parts used: Dried root.
• Dose: 1g per day.

## MOTHERWORT
Leonurus cardiaca

The Latin name refers to the leaves shaped like a lion's tail. It is a great calmer if tension is causing palpitations or sweats. It improves the circulatory system and is also used to relieve any menstrual and menopausal problems. Motherwort can also help to lower blood pressure.

**n o t e s** • Parts used: Leaves and flowers.
• Dose: 1 tsp dried/2 tsp fresh to a cup of boiling water three times a day, or 2 tsp syrup.
**c a u t i o n :** It is important that it is avoided in the first trimester of pregnancy.

## LEMON BALM
Melissa officinalis, Bee Balm

This plant has so much vitality that it can spread all over the garden. It makes a suitable drink for every day; hot in winter and iced in summer. Lemon Balm aids digestion and relaxation, and sensitive digestive systems. It is much used for irritable bowels, nervous indigestion, anxiety and depression. It makes a good bedtime drink, promoting peaceful sleep and a sense of relaxation.

**n o t e s** • Parts used: Leaves and flowers.
• Dose: 1 tsp to a cup of boiling water, taken up to three or four times a day.

## MINT
Mentha spp.

Peppermint (Mentha piperita) is a hybrid between Spearmint and Watermint. It is antiseptic and anti-parasitic, and will reduce itching. It has a temporary anaesthetic effect on the skin and gives the impression of cooling. It is included in lotions for massaging aching muscles, and makes an effective footbath.

**n o t e s** • Parts used: Leaves and flowers.
• Dose: 1 tsp dried/2 tsp fresh to a cup of boiling water.
**c a u t i o n :** It is important that it is avoided in the first trimester of pregnancy.

## EVENING PRIMROSE
Oenothera biennis

A beautiful plant, luminous in the twilight, which freely self-seeds in the garden. It is used externally for eczema and other dry skin conditions. Taken internally, Evening Primrose oil reduces cholesterol levels and benefits the circulation. It has a decent success rate on women with PMS, and can help calm hyperactive children. It also helps regenerate livers which have been damaged by alcohol.

**n o t e s** • Parts used: Oil from seeds.
• Dose: Capsules as directed.
**c a u t i o n :** Avoid in cases of epilepsy.

## MARJORAM
Origanum vulgare

There are many species of Marjoram, and they are used in potpourris and cooking. Medicinally, Marjoram reduces depression and helps tackle nervous headaches. It contains volatile oils which are antispasmodic, making it useful when soothing digestive upsets. The infused oil can be used in the bath to relieve stiffness, or rubbed on to soothe sore and aching joints or muscles.

**n o t e s** • Parts used: Leaves.
• Dose: I tsp dried/2 tsp fresh to a cup of boiling water, taken twice a day.

## PASSION FLOWER
Passiflora incarnata, Maypop

This is a climbing plant which produces spectacular flowers. It is often included in sleeping mixes, and is very helpful when tackling restlessness and insomnia. It counteracts the effects of adrenaline, which may cause anxiety, palpitations or nervous tremors. It is used to ease the pain of neuralgia.

**n o t e s** • Parts used: Dried leaves and flowers.
• Dose: ¼-½ tsp dried herb twice a day, or I tsp at night, or take an over-the-counter preparation as directed.

## ROSEMARY
Rosmarinus officinalis

A familiar plant containing several active, aromatic oils. Like Lavender, it can be used both externally, in the form of an essential or infused oil, and internally as a flavouring, tea or tincture. The actions of Rosemary are centred on the head and womb. It increases the supply of blood to both. In the head it helps tackle cold headaches and in the gut eases spasms due to poor circulation.

**n o t e s** • Parts used: Leaves and flowers.
• Dose: I tsp to a cup of boiling water taken up to three times a day.

## SAGE
Salvia officinalis

A beautiful, evergreen plant with fine purple flowers in early summer. Like many culinary herbs, it aids digestion. It has antiseptic properties and can be used as a compress on wounds that are slow to heal, or as a gargle or for infections of the mouth or throat. It is also said that it will help reduce night sweats and menopausal hot flushes, and can darken greyish hair.

**n o t e s** • Parts used: Leaves.
• Dose: I tsp dried per cup of boiling water.
**c a u t i o n :** Avoid during pregnancy.

## SKULLCAP
Scutellaria lateriflora

This herb is another nervous tonic. It was traditionally associated with the head, because it produces skull-like seed pods. It is very calming. Skullcap can help reduce anxiety and restlessness. Its bitter taste encourages the liver to remove toxins from the body, as well as excess hormones which can cause degrees of premenstrual tension.

**n o t e s** • Parts used: Aerial parts, which are harvested after flowering.
• Dose: I tsp dried/2 tsp fresh to a cup of boiling water.

## WOOD BETONY
Stachys betonica syn. S. officinalis, Betonica officinalis, Bishop's Weed

An attractive plant with purple flowers. Wood Betony aids the nervous system, especially if sick headaches and poor memory are a problem. It also encourages blood flow to the head. Always a popular remedy throughout Europe, it is certainly well worth trying if you get headaches or migraines.

**n o t e s** • Parts used: Aerial parts.
• Dose: I tsp dried/2 tsp fresh herb to a cup of boiling water.
**c a u t i o n :** It is important that you avoid high doses during pregnancy.

## LIME BLOSSOM

Tilia × europaea, Linden Blossom

The tall upstanding Lime tree has honey-scented blossom. Medicinally it is relaxing and cleansing. It makes a helpful tea for fevers and flu, especially if combined with Yarrow and Peppermint. It encourages sweating and aids the body through fevers. It is also used to reduce hardening of the arteries and high blood pressure, and to relieve migraines.

**n o t e s** • Parts used: Flowers, including the pale yellowish bracts.
• Dose: I tsp dried/2 tsp fresh to a cup of boiling water taken three times a day.

## DAMIANA

Turnera diffusa

Damiana grows in South America and the West Indies. It was previously called Turnera aphrodisiaca and is a tonic to the nervous and reproductive systems. It is useful if the sexual function is impaired. It is taken as a remedy by men, but the stimulant and tonic work equally well for women. Damiana is harvested when in flower, and is dried for use as an anti-depressant, and to relieve anxiety.

**n o t e s** • Parts used: Leaves and stem.
• Dose: 2 tsp to a cup of boiling water, which can be taken twice a day.

## VALERIAN

Valeriana officinalis, All Heal

This is a tall herb with whitish-pink flowers which grows in damp places. The root has a powerful sedative effect on the nervous system, and effectively reduces tension. It can be used to reduce period pains, spasms, palpitations, and hyperactivity. It is good if anxiety makes sleep difficult.

**n o t e s** • Parts used: Dried root.
• Dose: I tsp to a cup of boiling water at bedtime.
**c a u t i o n :** High doses taken over a long period may cause headaches.

## VERVAIN

Verbena officinalis, Herb of Grace

An unassuming plant with tiny flowers. Vervain is a nervous tonic with a slightly sedative action. It is useful for treating nervous exhaustion and symptoms of tension which include headaches, nausea and migraine. It has a bitter taste and has been used for gall bladder problems. It is quite often recommended for anyone who has depression, and works well with Wild Oats.

**n o t e s** • Parts used: Leaves and flowers.
• Dose: I tsp dried/2 tsp fresh to a cup of boiling water.

## CRAMP BARK

Viburnum opulus, Guelder Rose

A decorative wild bush which produces glorious white and pale pink spring flowers, followed by autumn red berries. Writer Geoffrey Grigson said it had a smell like crisply fried, well-peppered trout. Therapeutically, the use of Cramp Bark is a good illustration of the connection between body and mind. It reduces spasms whatever the cause and helps tackle constipation, period pains, and high blood pressure.

**n o t e s** • Parts used: Dried bark.
• Dose: I tsp to a cup of boiling water.

## CHASTE TREE

Vitex agnus-castus, Monk's Pepper

The common name reflects a slight anti-oestrogen effect which can cool passion: perhaps this property may account for its other common name, Monk's Pepper. Small doses of this herb can re-balance the hormones and reduce some of the symptoms of PMS, menopausal change, infertility, post-natal depression and irregular periods. It also increases milk production after birth.

**n o t e s** • Parts used: Dried ripe fruits.
• Dose: 10–20 drops of tincture which are taken first thing in the morning.

# homeopathy

homeopathy
homeopathy

The name "homeopathy" was coined by Samuel Hahnemann from two Greek words meaning "similar suffering", or "like cures like". Appalled by the savage medical practices of the day, Hahnemann, a German doctor and chemist, started on a course of study that led to the development of homeopathy. His philosophy of disease and its cure through natural processes has changed very little from that day to this. The traditional approach is today's approach.

The principle of like curing like, or "the law of similars", as it is sometimes called, decrees that if a substance can cause harm to a healthy person in large doses, it also has the potential to cure the same problem in tiny doses by stimulating the body's own natural energy, enabling it to heal itself.

The law is best illustrated by example. In the 19th century it was a custom among German women to take the herb Valerian as a stimulant. The practice was abused and overtaxed the nervous system. Yet, given in minute doses, Valerian relaxes the nervous system, and is one of homeopathy's main remedies for insomnia.

The doses used in homeopathy are so minute that they cannot be acting directly on the physical body. Hahnemann considered that what they did was act dynamically: in other words, the energy of the remedy stimulated the natural healing energy of the body. If it had been in a state of disharmony, then it would be propelled back to its former, healthy state.

# homeopathy and health

Homeopathy is not only an energy medicine, it is also holistic. Homeopaths convincingly argue that the body is much more than the sum of its various parts, and that the mind, the emotions and indeed the organs are somehow intricately interconnected. Consequently, the treatments they give are more "rounded" than those found in traditional medicine. They are not just aimed at the symptom, but at the whole person.

## ENERGY WITHIN

The mechanics of this interconnection are elaborate and hard to explain, but it is clear that the process really does work. The key point is that underlying the physical and mental systems of the body is a refined system of energy which is self-regulating. It generally works extremely well. You sense it in action when you become ill. We usually get better even without taking a medicine. The body heals itself though it might need support when its own natural energy is low.

### Treatment

The healing process is like running a car. Modern cars are so efficient that, provided you maintain them properly, give them the right fuel and drive them sensibly, problems seldom arise. Then one night you forget to turn off the lights and the next morning the battery is flat and your car incapacitated. The only way to get it moving again – the only cure – is to get a transfer of energy, in the form of a jump start from another battery. Homeopathy is in many ways just like getting an energizing jump start.

Homeopathy is becoming increasingly popular because of the serious concerns about drugs-based orthodox medicine. Many drugs are toxic and the side-effects in susceptible people can actually be quite unpleasant. Even if the side-effects are not observable, the long-term consequences from the excessive use of drugs are not always fully appreciated. In fact modern medicine seldom cures, and it does not even pretend to. What it does do is alleviate and palliate the symptoms, and manage the illness, but since it addresses the symptoms and rarely the cause, the results are not entirely satisfactory.

Homeopathy is different because it is safe and it does not treat the removal of symptoms as an end in itself. Symptoms are considered as signs of distress or adjustment. The correct remedy removes the cause of the problem; the symptoms will then fade away. Homeopathy is highly rated because it takes into account the nature of the person. It knows that when two people have been diagnosed as having the same illness, they can actually become ill in quite different ways and will require different remedies to effect a satisfactory cure.

*Sometimes our bodies just do not seem to be firing on all cylinders, and we need a carefully chosen homeopathic boost to revive them.*

## DEFINING DISEASE

We become ill when our energy is depleted or when we are out of harmony. In fact the word "disease" could be more accurately written "dis-ease", indicating that we are definitely not at ease, and for a disease to be cured it is not necessary to give it a name. To cure homeopathically depends on a sensitive, accurate analysis of the symptoms. There is usually no need for a diagnosis, for it is widely said that there are no diseases, only what might be called people who are "dis-eased".

### Symptoms

Except for any life-threatening situations, symptoms are not the primary problem. They reflect a picture which shows how the system is making adjustments to heal itself. For example, both diarrhoea and vomiting are the body's way of ridding itself of unwanted "material", and the intolerable itching of eczema does not specifically mean that you have a skin disease. Rather it means that there is an imbalance in your whole system, and that your body is pushing the problem to the safest possible place, well away from the essential organs. The skin becomes an organ of elimination.

### Treating the Whole Person

Some people are very robust and seldom become ill, others are over-sensitive and become run-down and sick after a slight chill or an emotional upset. For some, the chest is the greatest weakness: winter colds quickly turn to bronchitis. With others digestion is the problem: the slightest unusual change to their diet causes an immediate upset. Homeopathy acknowledges these many differences and adjusts all treatments accordingly. The professional homeopath will always prescribe "constitutionally" to try to strengthen the weak areas, as well as the whole system.

### Causes of Illness

There are many causes of disease. Some are obvious, such as being run-down and poor nutrition, but illness might have an emotional cause. Stress creates disharmony which manifests itself in physical ailments. Homeopathy takes such factors into account and, if possible, tries to mitigate them and strengthen the sufferer.

*Mental and emotional stress, often at work, can surprisingly quickly lead to a range of physical problems.*

## CHRONIC DISEASES

With so much battering from within and without, it may seem a wonder that we are not all permanently ill. Of course, many people are. Although many of the acute infectious diseases of the past have ceased to be a serious problem, their places have now been taken by today's chronic diseases. Never has there been so much cancer and heart disease, eczema and asthma, or even digestive problems such as irritable bowels. Our immune systems are overstretched in combating these problems.

### The Immune System

It is all too easy to ignore the incredible adaptability and intelligence of the immune system, which appears to make heroic efforts to keep us up and running despite considerable adversity. One writer shrewdly called this intelligence the "vital force". He described it as "the spirit-like force which rules in supreme sovereignty". It has also been well described as "the invisible driver", overseeing the checks and balances that are needed to keep us in the best possible health.

### The Vital Force at Work

Most of the time we are completely and utterly unaware of this sophisticated balancing process which is entirely automatic and pre-programmed through our genetic make-up. We can certainly observe it in action when we contract an acute illness (i.e. one that arises suddenly) such as a fever or a cough. What we may not always realize is that the fever is really a necessary, natural function and that it actually "burns up" the infection, and that the cough exists to prevent any active accumulation of mucus in the lungs. The body is extremely resourceful. However, chronic diseases (i.e. those that develop slowly, or are of long duration) might well need outside help, and a consultation with an experienced, professional practitioner.

## Reading the Symptoms

When trying to cure a disease, the vital force causes the body to produce symptoms. Homeopaths call this "the symptom picture". These symptoms accurately reflect exactly what is happening inside, and they also indicate what outside help or extra energy is therefore now required.

For example, during a flu epidemic two children in the same family become ill. The first child catches the flu very suddenly, overnight, and develops a high fever with a red face and a dry burning heat all over the body. The second child's symptoms might be very different, appearing quite slowly over several days. This child's fever is much lower, but he is shaky and shivery and his muscles ache all over. Both children have the same flu, but the vital force has produced completely different symptoms. Each child therefore needs to be treated in quite a different way. The homeopath will certainly understand this and give the first child the remedy Belladonna, while the second child receives quantities of Gelsemium. Homeopathy is well known for excelling at individualizing such treatments.

While it is quite true to say that in homeopathy we do not treat symptoms but the individual sufferer, we are still extremely interested in the symptoms. For it is through careful observation of the complete symptom picture that we can discover which remedy is required. In acute ailments the vital force will eventually effect a cure, given sufficient time, but by giving a helping hand from an accurate reading of the symptoms, that is by giving the body an "energy fix", the process can in fact be speeded up considerably.

*We are all born with a vital force that oversees our health.*

# using remedies

When first taking a homeopathic remedy, you might well be totally bewildered how anyone could possibly know that a certain recipe of mixed ingredients is the one that is best for you. In fact there is no guesswork. The exact remedies for all kinds of problems have been known and listed for hundreds of years. The technique is precise and proven, and the beauty of it is that remedies can be subtly fine-tuned to suit your particular ailment.

## REMEDY SOURCES

The remedies used in homeopathy are derived from many sources. The majority are prepared from plants, but many minerals are also used and a few remedies are even prepared from insect and snake poisons and other toxic substances. Do not be alarmed about the toxins because they have been diluted so that no danger remains. The Law of Similars shows that the most powerful poisons can be turned into equally strong remedies. In fact about 2,000 have now been described and documented, but in practice most professional homeopaths use only a fraction of that surprisingly high number.

*In homeopathy every symptom is fully taken into account when trying to apply the right remedy.*

The process that turns a substance into a remedy is called "potentization", and consists of two main procedures, dilution and succussion (or vigorous shaking). When you buy a remedy note a number after its name, usually 6, but also other numbers rising in a scale: 30, 200, 1M (1,000). Sometimes a "c", standing for centesimal (one hundredth) appears after the number. It shows how often the remedy has been diluted and succussed.

A remedy is prepared by dissolving a tincture of the original material, usually in alcohol. On the centesimal scale, the 6th potency means that the original substance has been diluted six times, each time using a dilution of one part in a hundred. This results in a remedy that contains only one part in a million million of the source material. Yet the greater the potency (number of dilutions), the greater the remedy's power.

Between each dilution, the remedy is succussed. When the potentization is complete the remedy is preserved in alcohol, and a few drops can be added to a bottle of milk-sugar pills or a cream. The remedy is now ready to use.

### Tissue Salts

The 19th-century German doctor Wilhelm Schussler identified 12 vital minerals, or "tissue salts", essential to health. According to his theory, many diseases are associated with a deficiency of one or more of these substances, but they can be cured by taking the tissue salts in minute doses, singly or in all kinds of different combinations.

## PROVINGS

Almost all homeopathic remedies have been "proved", or tested, although practitioners gain additional knowledge of them from clinical experience. In a proving, a remedy is tested on a group of healthy people over a period of time, until they develop symptoms. Neither the supervisor nor the group should know what remedy they are proving. This is a double blind test, conducted on sound, regulated principles. The symptoms that the provers develop are accurately collated until a complete symptom picture has been obtained. Consequently, we know exactly what the remedy can cure.

Once proved, remedies can be used for all time. Hundreds of original remedies are still in use today. The remedy pictures are described in great detail in volumes called *Materia Medica*. Because thousands of symptoms for thousands of remedies have been proved over the last 200 years or so, no one homeopath could possibly remember them all. They are therefore listed in another impressively detailed book called *The Homeopathic Repertory*. It is, in effect, an index to the *Materia Medica*. Between them, these two astonishing books cover most symptoms.

*In homeopathy, physical examinations are seldom necessary, but bright, sparkling eyes are a sign of good health.*

*Even members of the same family will have different susceptibilities to illness and react differently.*

## CHOOSING THE CORRECT REMEDY

With a copy of the *Materia Medica*, the homeopath is now well equipped to match the symptoms with the symptom picture. This is usually known as finding the similimum (or similar).

### The Symptom Picture

Finding the correct remedy is like trying to arrange a perfect marriage. If the two partners are compatible, success is almost certain. If the remedy is a good match to the symptoms, the patient is going to feel a good deal better, the natural way. The words "I feel better in myself" are like music to the ears of the prescribing homeopath, because it means that the natural healing processes have been stimulated successfully, even if some of the physical symptoms remain. It should be only a short time before they too disappear.

The prescriber is like a detective looking for clues. Apart from the obvious general symptoms, such as fever, headache or a cough, you should note what are called the "modalities" – that is, what aggravates or alleviates the symptoms, or makes the person feel generally better or worse. They might include the need for warmth, or cool air, sitting up or lying down. Notice whether the person is thirsty or sweaty; whether the tongue is coated, and the state of the breath. What kind of pain is it: throbbing, stitching or sudden stabs of intense agony?

It is also important to note if the symptoms have an obvious cause? Did they arise after an emotional shock, or after catching a chill in a cold wind? Did they arise dramatically and suddenly in the middle of the night, or have they developed in rather a nondescript way over a number of days?

It is also very important to note the person's state of mind. For example, irritable people who just want to be left alone may need quite different remedies from those who want to be comforted and are easily consoled. The homeopath has to be sensitive in all kinds of ways.

## HOW TO USE REMEDIES

Many minor and self-limiting acute problems can be treated safely at home with a basic first-aid kit. However, for more serious long-term ailments, or if you feel out of your depth and really worried – especially if young children or old people are ill – seek help from your own homeopath or doctor. Access to professional homeopaths is now much easier, and they can often do wonderful things for persistent and chronic disease. Be assured that qualified practitioners will have completed three or four years' training.

What the given remedy is doing is helping your body to help itself. Sometimes there may not be a great deal you can do – a well-established cold is going to mean several days of suffering whether you intervene or not. In other cases, the sooner you act, the better: for instance, if you take Arnica (either in pill form, or rubbed-in cream if appropriate) immediately after a bad fall for the bruising and shock, the results will be very impressive with the healing time being be much shorter.

You can often limit the duration or intensity of suffering, as in fever, sepsis (pus-forming bacteria), pain, indigestion and many other conditions. Moreover, there will be many satisfying times when the problem is aborted or cured altogether.

Once you are confident of an improvement then the vital force needs no further help, and you can stop taking the remedy. You will do no harm if you do in fact carry on, but there is really no point in trying to acquire far more energy than your mind and body actually require. In homeopathy it is perfectly true to say that less is actually more.

*You may feel rather hesitant and uncertain about treating very young children, but it is known that homeopathy usually works extremely well on them, and can be safely used from birth.*

remedies for common ailments
remedies for common ailments

# remedies for common ailments

Many straightforward problems can be treated at home using homeopathy. For each one, the following pages list a number of remedies that are likely to be the most helpful in the situation. Read the remedy picture carefully and choose the one that best seems to match the symptoms that you have observed. Then, when you have selected your own particular remedy, double-check it very carefully with the more detailed description which you will find listed in the Materia Medica section. Rescue Remedy is often used by homeopaths, though it is not strictly homeopathic, for that reason it has not been included in the Materia Medica.

## How to Take the Remedy

Carefully empty one pill into the cap of the bottle. If more than one tumbles into the cap, tip the others back into the bottle without touching them. This is quite important. If you are shaky, use a folded piece of paper to help if necessary.

Next, drop the pill on to a clean tongue – that is, you should take the remedy at least ten minutes before or after eating, drinking or cleaning your teeth. The pill should be sucked for about thirty seconds before being crunched and swallowed. Remedies for babies can be crushed to a powder in an envelope and given on a teaspoon.

## Giving the Remedy

The 6th and 30th potencies are most useful for home use. As a rough rule of thumb, use a 6c three or four times a day, or a 30c once or twice daily until symptoms improve. One pill at a time is all that is necessary; there is no need to reduce the dosage for children.

In serious situations such as a high fever or after an accident, you can give a remedy every half-hour if necessary. Since the active content of the remedy is so small, you cannot overdose in acute situations and if you do not get a good reaction within a day or overnight, you may want to consider a second remedy. Never worry about giving the wrong remedy: it will either work or it will not. If it does not work you will have done no harm to the patient.

Sometimes the symptoms may change after giving a remedy, so that a new picture emerges. You then need to find a new remedy to fit the new picture. If the situation improves, or the picture is unclear, watch and wait. Only intervene if you feel you need to.

Until you get used to the method of diagnosis, you may find it helpful to consult a practitioner on the first few occasions, this is also a good idea if symptoms persist. The Homeopath will also be able to give other effective advice.

# colds, flu and toothache

Most colds, unless nipped in the bud, take their natural course and they should clear up in about week. Even so, they can make life pretty uncomfortable, as can a throbbing toothache. Flu, however, can be much more debilitating, though a good remedy can often help ameliorate the symptoms, soon reducing the effects of aching bones, weak legs, headaches, high temperatures, shivering and even dizziness.

## Colds and Flu

If flu comes on suddenly, often at night and perhaps after catching a chill, with symptoms of high fever and profuse sweating, Aconite is a perfectly good remedy. If the symptoms are similarly sudden and with a high temperature, but accompanied by redness, burning heat and a headache, then the remedy is much more likely to be Belladonna.

For flu that appears more slowly, accompanied by extreme thirst, irritability and the desire to be left alone, Bryonia will be very useful. Probably the most widely used remedy in flu, though, is Gelsemium. The most pronounced symptoms are shivering, aching muscles and general weakness. Where aching bones are prominent, use Eupatorium.

For head colds with sneezing and an acrid nasal discharge, Allium cepa or Arsenicum should be very helpful. If the sinuses are also affected and there is a lot of yellow-green mucus which appears in globules, or if it looks sticky and stringy, then use quantities of Kali bich.

For a general tonic, both during and after the flu, when your symptoms are not very well defined and there is a general feeling of malaise, try using Ferrum phos.

*Kali bich can be a good remedy for blocked sinuses where there is pain and a green stringy discharge.*

*The most useful remedies at the start of a high fever in children are Aconite and Belladonna.*

## Fevers

Fevers, particularly in children, whose temperatures may be quite high, may seem alarming, but it should be remembered that they are the body's own efficient, natural response to dealing with and burning up infection.

The two main remedies for high fevers that appear suddenly are Aconite and Belladonna. Thirst and sweat characterize the Aconite picture, while Belladonna cases will reveal a dry skin, redness, and a throbbing pain in the affected area. If the fever appears more slowly and the person is irritable, wants to be left alone and is very thirsty for cold water, try Bryonia. For flu-like fevers, with shivering, weakness and aching muscles, use Gelsemium. Ferrum phos can be used in milder fevers, with no particularly distinctive symptoms. Pulsatilla is really useful in children's fevers, where the child soon becomes very emotional, clingy and weepy, and wants to be comforted.

If the period of fever is made more uncomfortable by poor circulation and chilblains, the former can be helped by herbs that stimulate the circulatory system. Angelica and Ginger have a good track record, taken with the likes of Yarrow. The latter is best treated by a tincture of Arnica.

*At the first sign of a head cold, try Arsenicum or Allium cepa.*

## Coughs and Croup

For very harsh, dry, violent coughs, which may appear suddenly and may be worse at night, use Aconite. For a hard, dry painful cough, which seems to be helped by holding the chest very tightly and also by long drinks of cold water, use Bryonia.

For deep-seated, dry, spasmodic coughs that may end in retching or even vomiting, use Drosera. Painful, barking coughs, which produce thick yellow-green mucus, may be helped by Hepar sulph. For coughs that are really quite suffocating, and which sound sharp and rasping, like a saw going through wood, try Spongia. Where there is a lot of mucus seemingly trapped in the chest, try Ant tart.

Croup is a horrible sounding dry cough that affects small children. The main remedies are Aconite, Hepar sulph and Spongia. Try each one of these remedies in turn if it is in any way difficult to differentiate between the symptoms.

## Sore Throats

If a sore throat starts suddenly, often during the night, perhaps following a chill and accompanied by a high temperature, try Aconite. If the throat burns and throbs painfully and looks very red, it may be eased by Belladonna.

For a sore throat that looks very swollen and puffy, with a stinging pain, try Apis. Hepar sulph can be used for an extremely painful throat that feels as if there is a fish bone stuck in it, making it very difficult to try and swallow.

If the sore throat feels worse on the left side and swallowing liquids is particularly painful, use Lachesis. Use Lycopodium if the throat is worse on the right side or the pain moves from right to left; warm drinks may be comforting.

For a sore throat which is accompanied by offensive breath and saliva, with a degree of sweatiness and thirst, then you should try Mercurius. For throats that appear dark, raw and red, and feel as if a highly uncomfortable, unpleasant hot lump has got stuck inside, try taking quantities of Phytolacca. That usually proves quite effective.

## Relieving Toothache

There is probably no worse agony than the pain of toothache, as the area is so sensitive. In most cases, a visit to the dentist will be essential, but the following remedies may well help you cope with the pain in the meantime.

For sudden and violent pains, perhaps precipitated by a cold, Aconite may be helpful. If the area looks very red and throbs violently, Belladonna should be used. For abscesses, where pus is obviously present and the saliva tastes and smells foul, the best remedy is likely to be Mercurius. If you are prone to abscesses and your teeth are generally not very strong, Silica should be used to strengthen the system.

For pain that lingers after a visit to the dentist, take Arnica or Hypericum. If the pain is in any way accompanied by extreme irritability, Chamomilla should be used.

Hepar sulph is a suitable remedy for extreme septic states (infected areas), where bad temper is a prominent symptom. Another remedy for toothache where there are spasmodic shooting pains is Mag phos.

*Though there are several remedies that can help with toothache, you will still need to visit the dentist.*

# eyes and ears
Any problems with the eyes and ears can be immediately quite distressing, especially for young children who do not appreciate what is happening. Their world can suddenly be turned upside down. Fortunately, there is a wide range of proven remedies for helping ease such discomfort, for example reducing puffy, swollen eyes, styes, burning sensations, and even the debilitating effects of a sudden, throbbing ear infection.

## SOOTHING THE EYES
Overwork, pollutants, viral and bacterial infections can all affect the delicate tissues in and around the eyes. Stress and fatigue tend to aggravate these problems by weakening the immune system's ability to fight off infection.

Aconite helps when the eye feels hot and dry, perhaps after catching a cold. The eye may feel irritated, as if it has got a piece of grit. Apis is a good remedy to use when the eyelids look puffy and swollen; the discomfort can be reduced and relieved by applying a cold compress.

Belladonna is a very good remedy for eyes that look in any way red and bloodshot, and which are over-sensitive to light. Euphrasia is one of the very best remedies for sore and burning eyes, and it can also be used in an eyebath because it can be obtained in a diluted tincture.

One of the best remedies for styes is Pulsatilla, which should be used when the eye has an infection which results in what is best described as a sticky yellow discharge. When treating eye injuries, Symphytum can be used where there has been a blow to the eyeball. For general eye injuries, Arnica will ease the bruising. Ledum helps when the eye is cold and puffy.

*Eye irritants cause a lot of discomfort and need tackling quickly.*

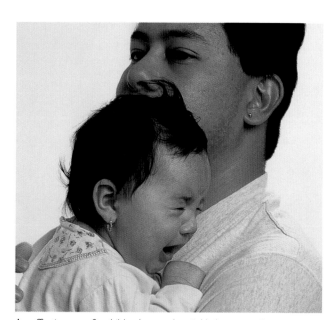

*An effective cure for children's earaches is Verbascum oil.*

## EAR INFECTIONS
Acute earaches are most common in young children. They need to be treated quickly, as an infection within the middle ear can be both painful and damaging. Speedy home help can be very useful, but you must get professional medical help if the earache worsens or if it in any way persists.

One of the most soothing remedies is Verbascum oil. Pour a few drops into a spoon that has been pleasantly warmed, and drip gently into the child's ear.

For sudden and violent pains, accompanied by fever which usually start at night, use Aconite. Where there is a fever with a sudden and violent appearance, and the ear throbs and looks very red, Belladonna will effect a cure.

For earaches where there is great pain and the child is exceptionally irritable, use Chamomilla. Ferrum phos is required where the pain comes on slowly and there are no other significant distinguishing symptoms. For very painful, sore earaches with some discharge of yellow-green mucus, when the child is also clearly chilly and irritable, use Hepar sulph.

# allergies

Over the last 20 or 30 years there has been a highly significant increase in all kinds of allergies, which might be better described as the body's sensitivity to an excess of substances that cannot be easily assimilated. Sadly, many such substances are the product of our time. Hay fever, eczema, asthma, irritable bowel disease and other chronic diseases have now reached almost epidemic proportions. Fortunately, homeopathy can offer you essential help.

## HAY FEVER

Hay fever is rather a misnomer, for there are many other substances apart from hay which can trigger the well-known symptoms of watering eyes and runny nose, itchiness and sneezing. The problem may last for a few weeks, a few months or even all year, depending on the cause.

Euphrasia and Allium cepa are two of the most effective acute remedies. If the problem is centred in the eyes, with even the tears burning, Euphrasia is the remedy to use. However, if the nasal symptoms are worse, with constant streaming and an acrid discharge, then try Allium cepa. Another remedy that is sometimes useful when there are constant burning secretions from the mucous membranes is Arsenicum.

To build up your immune system, it is best to act about two to three months before the time when hay fever usually begins. There are plenty of tasty aids. Garlic, in pill form or meals when it can even be eaten whole if roasted in the oven, imparting a new, sweetish flavour, works well. So too do regular applications of honey. Inhaling over a steam bath using lemon balm reduces the chances of an allergic attack.

*Red onion, the source of the remedy,* Allium cepa.

## CHRONIC DISEASES

No one knows precisely what causes these problems. Further research is required. Quite clearly there are many different reasons. Toxicity overload is almost certainly one. The body simply cannot cope with the increasingly large number of chemicals and drugs that it was never designed to absorb. Another likely reason is deficient nutrition. Many of our foods are now so over-processed (apart from being sprayed with all kinds of chemicals) that they do not contain sufficient minerals and vitamins to allow the body to function efficiently.

Homeopathy can often work wonders in correcting the many weaknesses that result from such causes. Obviously, you should also take care to avoid toxic substances wherever possible, and eat a healthy, varied diet. The homeopathy that is needed to cure chronic ailments is complex and beyond the scope of this book; seek advice from a professional homeopath.

*Allergies, or over-sensitivity to certain foods, are becoming increasingly common. Research shows that dairy products and wheat-based foods seem to cause the most problems.*

# acute illnesses and upsets

There is nothing quite as frustratingly disabling as a sudden upset stomach, whether it be diarrhoea, lingering indigestion, niggling cramps or even quite painful bouts of trapped wind. But with the use of homeopathy you do not have to keep on suffering. It actually offers several well-proven ways of helping you tackle such problems, so that you can resume a normal life, quickly getting out and about.

## SETTLING GASTRIC UPSETS

The main symptoms of stomach and intestinal infections are pain, wind (gas), nausea, vomiting and diarrhoea. Bear in mind that vomiting and diarrhoea are actually natural processes by which the body rids itself quickly of any unwanted material. Consequently these symptoms need to be treated only if they are persistent. Such problems can arise at any time and may be due to food poisoning or just a sudden reaction to unfamiliar food; this invariably seems to happen on vacation.

### Upset Stomach

The great standby remedy is Arsenicum. Other symptoms which may accompany diarrhoea or vomiting are excessive weakness, coldness and restlessness. Mag phos is an excellent remedy for general abdominal cramps which are soothed by doubling up and making sure that you keep warm.

For constant nausea which is unrelieved by vomiting, use Ipecac. Nux vomica is a very good remedy for gastric upsets where nothing really seems to happen. The undigested food lies like a horrible dead weight in the stomach and refuses to move or be expelled, causing plenty of discomfort.

Phosphorus can be a useful remedy for diarrhoea, and it is particularly effective if attacks are accompanied by a sensation of burning in the stomach. While you may crave a cold drink, it is actually vomited as soon as it warms up in the stomach.

*A piece of Arsenopyrite used in the remedy Arsenicum.*

### Indigestion

The symptoms of indigestion are heartburn, wind (gas) and cramping pains. They are usually caused by eating too much or in fact eating too quickly. The symptoms are usually much more marked when you are eating very rich food and drinking large quantities of alcohol. The most useful remedy is Nux vomica. The digestive system seems heavy and sluggish and the feeling is that you would be much better if the undigested food would move. Another good remedy that can help is Lycopodium.

## CALMING BOILS AND ABSCESSES

Sometimes, an area of skin becomes inflamed and gathers pus. This usually happens around a hair follicle. The build-up of pus can cause acute pain before it comes to a head as a boil or abscess, or until the pus is absorbed by the body.

In the early stages of a boil or abscess, when it looks red and angry and throbs painfully, Belladonna is often the best remedy. Later when it starts becoming septic (infected) and even more painful as the pus increases, use Hepar sulph. If the boil seems very slow in coming to a head, Silica should be used to speed up the process. This remedy is also helpful as a daily tissue salt for unhealthy skin that keeps producing boils. The nails may also be unhealthy, breaking and peeling too easily.

*Belladonna is highly effective against a wide range of complaints.*

# emotional issues

We underrate at surprisingly great risk the incredible part that our emotions can play in our health. Diseases can easily arise from any disharmony in our lives. This is even more likely if we are repressed, unable to express and articulate our more difficult, upsetting emotions, feelings staying trapped and locked within us. Just as joy can bolster and keep us in good health, a big build-up of grief can result in all kinds of illness.

## Emotional Turmoil

It is not unusual for a homeopathic practitioner to hear words like "I've never really got over my father's death," or "I've never properly felt well since my divorce." It is important for good health not to allow such wounds to fester. Homeopathy can often help chronic and acute conditions when needed.

In any emotional situation where you feel that you really cannot cope, the Bach Flower Rescue Remedy is useful. Although it is not strictly homeopathic, it works well with homeopathic remedies, and can be taken as often as you wish.

## Grief and Fright

Ignatia is the number-one remedy for acute feelings of sadness and loss. It can calm both the hysterical and over-sensitive and those who tend to keep their grief bottled up. Children and emotionally dependent people can be helped by Pulsatilla. Aconite is considered the major remedy for helping people who need to get over a shock or a terrifying experience.

## Anticipation

The worry brought on by a forthcoming event such as an exam, appearing on the stage or meeting someone new can severely affect some people. Fortunately, there are a number of remedies that can help ease any anxiety and panic.

*The most useful remedy for dealing with emotional upsets is Pulsatilla, combined with plenty of security and love.*

Gelsemium is best used when you start trembling with nerves and literally go weak at the knees. Arg nit is a good all-round anxiety remedy, where there are symptoms of great restlessness. It also has a claustrophobic picture and could help those who suffer from a fear of flying or even travelling on underground trains. The panic often causes diarrhoea, and another anxiety remedy that can help the bowels is called Lycopodium. Strangely, people who need Lycopodium are often found to excel at the ordeals that they have been worrying about, once they have overcome the panic barrier.

## Insomnia

There can be many causes of sleeplessness including worry, habit, and bad eating. For the "hamster on the wheel" syndrome, where your mind is rushing around in never-ending circles, Valerian can be a magical aid helping you quickly fall asleep. For those sufferers who constantly wake too early, especially if they are people who live too much on their nerves and eat large quantities of rich food, try Nux vomica.

*A Pasque flower, used in Pulsatilla.*

# women's health

Two of the greatest concerns to most women are their reproductive systems and the effects of their associated hormones, but many find they are treated in quite a heavy-handed way by traditional modern medicine. Fortunately, homeopathy offers another route and a range of different treatments which can include important aspects of your diet. Homeopathic self-help can ease the distress for various non-persistent conditions.

## Anaemia

Anaemia is usually caused by an iron deficiency and manifests itself through weakness, pallor and lack of stamina. The most vulnerable times are during pregnancy or after excessive blood loss due to heavy periods. Since iron pills supplied by your doctor can often severely upset the bowels, gentler methods are actually preferable. Eat foods rich in iron and try organic iron preparations which can be obtained from health food shops. Ferrum phos should also be used on a daily basis.

## Cystitis

Many women are familiar with the burning agony of urinating when they have a bladder infection. Cranberry juice or sodium bicarbonate can often help. Two of the most useful remedies are Cantharis and Apis. Use Cantharis as a general remedy. Apis can be helpful when the last drops in urination hurt the most.

## Mastitis

Mastitis means an inflammation of the breast and it occurs commonly during breast-feeding. It can be painful but is not normally serious. Fortunately, breast-feeding does not have to stop because of it. Homeopathy is usually very successful in curing the inflammation. Phytolacca is the most important remedy aiding breasts that may feel lumpy and swollen.

*A good diet is essential for good health. Fresh organic apples and other fruit are especially good for you.*

*PMT mood swings are not uncommon and should not alarm you. Check your symptoms to find a remedy that might help.*

## Pre-menstrual Syndrome (PMS)

Most women are familiar with the mood changes that arise just before an oncoming period. For an unfortunate few, more extreme symptoms of depression, anger and weepiness can appear, sometimes as much as a week or more before the flow begins. A visit to a professional homeopath can certainly be of great benefit, but there are several remedies that you might like to try yourself at home in order to alleviate some of these sudden, extreme symptoms.

Pulsatilla is an excellent remedy if weeping and the feeling of neediness is prominent. Sepia should be used where there is anger and exhaustion, and even in cases of indifference towards your family. Lachesis is very helpful in minimizing the more extreme symptoms of violent anger, jealousy and suspicion.

## Period Pains

If your period pains are consistently bad, you will need to consult a homeopath. For occasional pains, there are a number of self-help remedies from which you can choose. The three PMS remedies mentioned above, Pulsatilla, Sepia and Lachesis, should be considered when applicable, and if your symptoms seem significant and over-riding. All three might also be of some help during a difficult menopause.

# children's health
Children tend to respond very well and quickly to all kinds of homeopathic treatments, and they are a joy to treat. However, while there is actually no substitute for constitutional treatment from a professional homeopath who will try to boost the immune system as much as possible, there is no reason why you should not keep a good stock of remedies at home in case of a sudden, acute situation. You too can do a lot to help.

## Children and Homeopathy
The best start you can possibly give a child is plenty of confidence, with love and security, breast milk for as long as is practical, a healthy, varied diet, as few drugs as possible, and homeopathy. Young children invariably have rather dramatic, acute conditions, such as fevers. Usually there is nothing for you to worry about if you are well informed, have professional support and have access to remedies. The dosage is the same as for adults, but remember to crush the pills first for babies.

## Teething
The most widely used remedies for teething pains are Chamomilla and Pulsatilla. Chamomilla is an "angry" remedy and suits bad-tempered babies best. These are the ones that drain you of sympathy because you have had so many sleepless nights making you feel irritable and guilty for becoming bad tempered, and helpless. Only constant attention, picking them up and carrying them round, soothes them in any way. Pulsatilla children respond differently – they are softer, weepy and are constantly in need of your sympathy. They feel better and are significantly soothed by being given plenty of cuddles.

*For babies, it is essential to crush the tablet first.*

*Give your child the right start with love and a healthy diet.*

## Fevers
Many small children get fevers with very high temperatures, as they burn up infection in the most efficient way. Seek help if the fever goes on for more than 24 hours, especially if there are any signs at all of a violent headache or drowsiness. Aconite and Belladonna are the best, general high-fever remedies.

## Croup
This harsh, dry cough is very disturbing in small children, but usually sounds far worse than it really is. There are three main remedies for croup. Aconite can be used for particularly violent and sudden coughs, which are often worse at night. For harsh coughs that sound like sawing through wood, Spongia is the remedy. For a rattly chest with thick yellow-green mucus, possibly marked by irritability and chilliness, use Hepar sulph.

## Colic
Trapped wind can be very upsetting for a baby. It comes without warning, and for no apparent reason the baby will cry. Sometimes babies try to curl up to ease the pain, and warmth and a gentle massage should help. Mag phos is a useful remedy to try.

# first aid
Homeopathic remedies are extremely useful as first-aid treatments in all kinds of situations, but dangerous, serious injuries should always receive immediate, expert medical attention. If you are in any way alarmed or concerned, you must first call for help, at which point it might just be possible to start giving an appropriate remedy. In more minor cases, such as bruising, cuts and sprains, homeopathy can certainly make quite a difference.

## Bruises
The very first remedy to think of after any injury or accident is Arnica. For local bruising, where the skin is unbroken, apply Arnica cream, and whether you use the cream or not you can give an Arnica pill as often as you think necessary, until such time as the bruising starts to go down.

Arnica is also wonderful in cases of shock. If the person is dozy or woozy, or in fact unconscious, crush the remedy first and place the powder directly on to the lips.

Where there is serious shock, or in any real emergency, use Rescue Remedy. This can be used either alone or with Arnica in cases of physical trauma. Place a few drops of the Rescue Remedy straight on to the lips or tongue, every few minutes if considered necessary. If the injury results in pains shooting up the arms or legs, try using Hypericum.

This remedy is also very useful where sensitive areas have been injured and hurt, such as the toes, fingers, lips and ears. If the joints or bones have been hurt, Ruta may be more effective than Arnica, which is more of a soft tissue remedy.

## Cuts, Sores and Open Wounds
Clean the area thoroughly to remove all dirt. If the wound is deep, it may need stitches and you must seek instant medical help. Once the wound is clean, apply some Calendula cream.

*For bites that come up as any kind of bruise, small or dramatic, apply Arnica cream. For many it is very effective.*

*Calendula cream is a widely available, excellent remedy to use if you have got any open cuts and sores.*

## Puncture Wounds
Such injuries can easily occur in all kinds of ways: from animal or insect bites, pins, needles and nails, and even from standing on a sharp instrument such as a garden fork or rake.

If the wound becomes puffy and purple and feels cold, with the pain being eased by a cold compress, Ledum is the best remedy. If there are shooting pains, which travel up the limbs along the tracks of the nerves, then Hypericum should be used.

## Sprains, Strains and Fractures
For general muscle strains, resulting from lifting heavy weights or excessive physical exercise such as aerobics or long hikes over hilly countryside, Arnica will almost always be extremely effective. For deeper injuries where the joints are affected, as a result of a heavy fall or a strong football tackle, use Ruta.

For even more severe sprains, especially to the ankles or wrists, where the pain is agony on first moving the joint but eases with gentle limbering up, Rhus tox should be very helpful. For injuries where the slightest movement is extremely painful and hard pressure eases the pain, Bryonia will provide relief.

Once a broken bone has been set, use Symphytum daily, night and morning, for at least three weeks. This will not only ease the pain but speed up the healing of the bones.

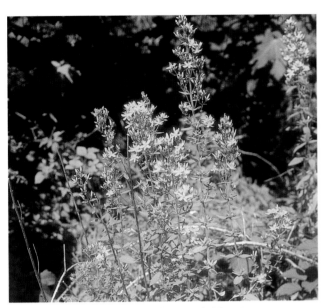

*The herb St John's Wort, used in the remedy Hypericum.*

## Burns

Severe burns need urgent medical assistance: do not delay, especially in the case of children and babies. For minor burns and scalds, Calendula or Hypercal cream can be very soothing, especially if applied straight away. If the pain remains, or the burn is severe, take one pill of the remedy Cantharis every few hours until the pain eases. In the case of shock or a hysterical child, also use Arnica (in pill form) and/or Rescue Remedy.

## Bites and Stings

For minor injuries, you can apply Calendula or Hypercal cream. If the wound looks in any way bruised, use Arnica, either as a cream or in pill form. However, if the wound becomes dramatically swollen and starts looking red and puffy, then use Apis. For any injuries to quite sensitive areas, such as the fingers, especially when shooting pains can be felt, Hypericum is a useful remedy. Ledum is preferable if the wound looks puffy and feels cold to the touch, and is helped by the application of a cold compress.

## Travel Sickness

Many people end up getting seasick even when the waves are not too rough, and some, especially children, are also air-sick or car-sick. The symptoms are eased by the remedy Cocculus.

## Fear of Flying

Use Aconite and/or Rescue Remedy before you go to the airport and then as often as you need during the flight. If you actually find yourself shaking with anxiety, try Gelsemium. If the problem is more a question of claustrophobia, the fear of being trapped in a narrow space, Arg nit should be very useful.

## Visits to the Doctor or Dentist

For any pre-visit nerves, to which we are all prone at some time, take Arg nit. For surgery or dental work where bruising and shock to the system might well have been involved, you cannot go wrong with Arnica. Take one pill before the treatment, and one pill three times a day for as long as you actively need it.

---

### The Homeopathic First-aid Kit

It is a good idea to keep a basic first-aid kit in the house so that you are well prepared for any sudden emergency. Many remedies are now available from health food shops and even some chemists, but for many of us there might not be a nearby source, and it is amazing how many emergencies arise outside shop-opening hours. Stock up and be safe.

**Your first-aid kit should include:**
Arnica cream – for bruises
Calendula cream – for cuts and sores
Echinacea tincture – for the immune system
Rescue Remedy tincture – for major emergencies

Although not strictly a homeopathic treatment, Rescue Remedy is one of Dr Edward Bach's Flower Remedies. These flower essences are a series of gentle plant remedies which are intended to treat various emotional states, regardless of the physical disorder.

**Plus these bottles of pills:**
Aconite – for fevers, coughs and colds
Apis – for bites and stings
Arnica – for bruising or shock following accidents
Arsenicum – for digestive upsets and food poisoning
Belladonna – for high fever and headaches
Bryonia – for dry coughs and fevers
Chamomilla – for teething and colic
Ferrum phos – for colds, flu and anaemia
Gelsemium – for flu and anxiety
Hepar sulph – for sore throats and infected wounds
Hypericum – for injuries

Ignatia – for grief and emotional upsets
Ledum – for puncture wounds, bites and stings
Lycopodium – for anxiety and digestive problems
Mercurius – for sepsis
Nux vomica – for hangovers, nausea and indigestion
Phosphorus – for digestive problems and nosebleeds
Pulsatilla – for ear infections, fevers and eye problems
Rhus tox – for sprains, strains and rashes
Ruta – for injuries to tendons and bones

# the materia medica

There are something like 2,000 remedies in the homeopathic Materia Medica, though most of them are actually best left to the professional practitioner. However, there are a surprising number of remedies that can safely be used by the lay person in low potencies for acute and first-aid cases. These remedies cover a wide range of not too serious, non-persistent problems. It is well worth seeing just how much you can achieve.

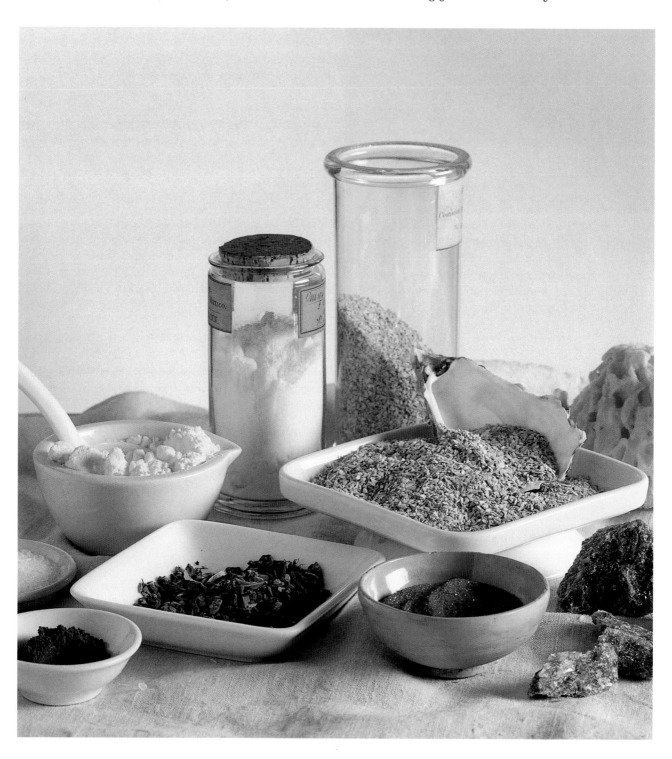

# HOMEOPATHIC CURES

Use this section to back up and confirm your choice from the remedies that were recommended for ailments earlier in the chapter on herbs. If your choice still looks good, then you are almost certainly on the right track. However, if it does not, then consider trying one of the other remedies which are described for the ailment. Do note, though, that not every particular symptom of the remedy has to be present. Homeopaths use the expression "a three-legged stool"; if the remedy covers three symptoms of the condition, then it is more than likely to be well indicated.

Note that you must always keep your supply of remedies in a cool, dark place or cupboard. Also do keep them well away from any strong, pervasive smells and young children. Fortunately, homeopathic remedies are known to be extremely safe, so even if a child does actually swallow a number of pills, even as much as a whole bottle, you need not be unduly alarmed or concerned.

# ACONITE
Aconitum napellus

Monkshood, a beautiful yet poisonous plant with blue flowers, is native to mountainous areas of Europe and Asia. It is widely cultivated as a garden plant.

**n o t e s** • Symptoms appear suddenly and violently, often at night. • They may appear after catching a chill or after a fright. • Fear or extreme anxiety may accompany symptoms. • An important remedy for high fevers with extreme thirst and sweat. • Major remedy for violent, dry croupy coughs. • It is most effective when used at the beginning of an illness.

# ALLIUM CEPA
Allium cepa

The remedy comes from the onion, whose characteristics are perfectly well known and obvious to anyone who has ever had to peel a strong one: it directly affects the mucous membranes of the nose, the eyes and throat.

**n o t e s** • Sneezing, often repeatedly, accompanied by a streaming nose. • The nose and eyes begin to burn and become irritated. • Nasal discharge is acrid while the tears are bland. • Major remedy for hay fever (when the nose is affected more than the eyes) and also for colds.

# ANT TART
Antimonium tartaricum

Ant tart is prepared from the chemical substance antimony potassium tartrate, and is traditionally referred to as tartar emetic. Ant tart affects the mucous membranes of the lungs.

**n o t e s** • A wet, rattling cough from deep in the lungs, with shortness of breath and wheezing. • Helps to bring up mucus from the lungs.

# APIS
Apis mellifica

The remedy is prepared from the honey bee. The well-known effects of its sting describe the remedy picture very well.

**n o t e s** • A useful remedy after injuries, especially from bites or stings where there is subsequent swelling, puffiness and redness. • The affected area feels like a water bag. • A fever appears quickly and without any thirst. • The person appears restless and irritable. • The symptoms are often relieved by the application of a cold compress, or exposure to cold air.

# ARG NIT
Argentum nitricum

Silver nitrate, from which this remedy is derived, is one of the silver compounds that are used during the photographic process. It is good at helping to soothe an agitated nervous system.

**n o t e s** • Panic, nervousness and anxiety. • Feeling worried, hurried and without emotional and practical support. • Fears of anticipation which might include stage fright, exams, visiting the dentist, flying, and many others. • The nervousness may cause diarrhoea and wind (gas).

## ARNICA
Arnica montana

Arnica is a well-known herb with yellow, daisy-like flowers. Its native habitat is mountainous areas. It has a special affinity with soft tissue and muscles, and is usually the first remedy to consider after any accident. Where there is bruising but the skin is not broken, use Arnica cream. (When the skin is broken, use Calendula or Hypercal cream.)

**n o t e s** • The most important remedy for bruising. • Shock following an accident. • Muscle strains after strenuous or extreme exertion.

## ARSENICUM
Arsenicum album

Arsenic oxide is a well-known poison. However, when used as a homeopathic remedy it is extremely safe and works especially well on the gastro-intestinal and respiratory systems.

**n o t e s** • Vomiting, diarrhoea, abdominal and stomach cramps. • Often the first remedy in cases of food poisoning. • Asthmatic, wheezy breathing, often worse at night. Head colds with a runny nose. • Chilliness, restlessness, anxiety and weakness. • Warmth gives great relief.

## BELLADONNA
Atropa belladonna

The valuable remedy Belladonna must be prepared from deadly nightshade, whose poisonous berries are best avoided. However, they produce a medicine which is one of the most important fever and headache remedies.

**n o t e s** • Violent and intense symptoms appearing suddenly. • Fever with high temperature, little thirst and burning, dry skin. • The face or the affected part is usually bright red. •Throbbing pains, especially in the head. •The pupils may be sensitive to light.

## BRYONIA
Bryonia alba

Bryonia is prepared from the roots of white bryony, a climbing plant which is found in hedgerows right across Europe. The roots are surprisingly large and store a great deal of water. Bryonia patients often seem to lack "lubrication".

**n o t e s** • The symptoms tend to develop slowly. • Dryness marks all symptoms: in the mouth, membranes and joints. • Extreme thirst. • The condition feels worse with the slightest motion.• Bryonia coughs are dry and very painful. • The person is irritable.

## CALENDULA
Calendula officinalis

Calendula has long been known to herbalists as a major first-aid remedy for injuries. It is prepared from the common marigold, and the simplest way to use it is as a cream. When combined with Hypericum it is known as Hypercal.

**n o t e s** • Use this cream on all cuts, sores and open wounds. (For bruises where the skin is not broken, use Arnica cream.) • Calendula is a natural antiseptic and keeps the injury free of infection, as well as helping to speed up the healing process.

## IPECAC
Cephaelis ipecacuanha

Ipecacuanha is a seemingly small, insignificant South American shrub. The remedy works mainly on the digestive and respiratory tracts, and the most important symptom it treats is nausea, no matter what the ailment.

**n o t e s** • Persistent nausea, not helped by vomiting. • Coughs that are accompanied by feelings of nausea. • Outbreaks of morning sickness during pregnancy. • Asthma or wheeziness accompanied by degrees of nausea. • Development of "sick" headaches.

## COCCULUS
Cocculus orbiculatus

The remedy is prepared from the Indian cockle, a plant that grows along the coasts of India. It profoundly affects the nervous system and can strengthen a weakened and exhausted system. Because it can also cure nausea and dizziness, it is considered an important remedy for all kinds of travel sickness, whether on a boat, plane or in a car.

**n o t e s** • Nausea, vomiting, and dizziness, as in travel sickness.
• Exhaustion and nervous stress, perhaps due to lack of sleep.

## DROSERA
Drosera rotundifolia

Drosera is a remedy prepared from an extraordinary insectivorous plant, the round-leaved sundew. The plants are often called "flypapers" because the leaves are tipped with sticky glands. The insect prey gets more embroiled the more it struggles, and is finally dissolved. Drosera affects the respiratory system and is an important cough remedy.

**n o t e s** • Deep, barking coughs.
• Prolonged and incessant coughs returning in periodic fits or spasms.
• The cough may result in retching.

## EUPATORIUM
Eupatorium perfoliatum

Eupatorium is a North American herb found growing in marshy places. It is used as a herb as a flu remedy, to lower fevers and even relieve congestion and constipation, as well as boosting the immune system. Its common name, boneset, gives a clue to its homeopathic use. Whatever the other symptoms, the bones usually do ache.

**n o t e s** • Flu-like symptoms, with aching all over, but pains that seem to have lodged deep in the bones.
• There may be a painful cough.

## EUPHRASIA
Euphrasia officinalis

Also known as eyebright, Euphrasia has long been known as a remedy with a specific application to the eyes. It is a very pretty little meadow plant, much used in wild flower plantings, with colourful flowers that open wide only when there is direct sunshine.

**n o t e s** • Eyes that are sore, red and inflamed. • The eyes water with burning tears. • In cases of hay fever, the symptoms are sneezing, itching and a runny nose, but for most the eyes are most usually affected.

## FERRUM PHOS
Ferrum phosphoricum

Iron phosphate, from which Ferrum phos is prepared, is a highly valued mineral that manages to balance the iron and oxygen in the blood. It is also a tissue salt and can be used actively as a tonic for anaemic patients who are beginning to feel rather weak and feeble.

**n o t e s** • Flu and cold symptoms that are not well defined.
• Weakness and tiredness. • General anaemia: the remedy can be very useful for women with heavy periods or during pregnancy.

## GELSEMIUM
Gelsemium sempervirens

The remedy is prepared from a North American plant known as yellow jasmine. It acts specifically on the muscles, the motor nerves and the nervous system. It is also quite probably the most important acute remedy for helping to treat an attack of flu.

**n o t e s** • Aching, heavy muscles which will not obey the will.
• Tiredness, weakness, shivering and trembling. • Fever with sweating but little thirst. • Headaches concentrated at the back of the head.

## HEPAR SULPH
Hepar sulphuris calcareum

The remedy was developed by Samuel Hahnemann, the first homeopath, from calcium sulphide, which is made by heating flowers of sulphur and the lime of oyster shells together. It strongly affects the nervous system and is good in acute septic states (infected areas) and in respiratory system problems.

**n o t e s** • Extreme irritability and over-sensitivity. • Coldness, especially around the head. • Hoarse, dry coughs with yellow mucus, croup. • Evidence of unusually heavy sweating.

## HYPERICUM
Hypericum perforatum

Prepared from the herb St John's Wort, Hypericum is primarily an injury remedy. It is particularly effective on any areas that have an abundant supply of sensitive nerves. They include the fingers, toes, lips, ears, eyes, and the coccyx at the base of the spine. Apply Hypericum instead of Arnica for bruising in such sensitive areas, although Arnica may work perfectly well if Hypericum is not available.

**n o t e s** • Pains are often felt suddenly shooting up the limbs, travelling along the tracks of the nerves.

## IGNATIA
Ignatia amara

Ignatia is prepared from the seeds of a tree, the St Ignatius bean, which grows in South-east Asia. It is well known as a major "grief" remedy, and it can strongly affect the emotions.

**n o t e s** • Sadness and grief following emotional loss. • Sudden changeable moods: tears following laughter, or hysteria. • Suppressed emotions, when the tears will not flow. • Pronounced bouts of sighing following a period of emotional unhappiness, particularly anxiety, fear or grief.

## KALI BICH
Kali bichromicum

The source of Kali bichromicum, potassium dichromate, is a chemical compound involved in many industrial processes which include dyeing, printing and photography. It especially affects the mucous membranes of the air passages, and is an important sinusitis remedy.

**n o t e s** • Highly unpleasant thick, strong, lumpy green discharges from the nasal passages or mouth. • Headaches in small spots as a result of catarrh. • Dry cough accompanied by sticky, yellow-green mucus.

## LACHESIS
Lachesis muta

Lachesis is prepared from the venom of the bushmaster snake which is native to South America. It is a chronic remedy best left to expert, professional homeopaths, but it does have an acute use when treating sore throats and also various menstrual problems.

**n o t e s** • Sore throats, much worse on the left side. • Painful throats where liquids are more difficult to swallow than solids. • Menstrual pains and tension improve when the flow starts. • Hot flushes around the menopause.

## LEDUM
Ledum palustre

The small shrub known as marsh tea, from which Ledum is derived, grows in boggy places across the cold wastes of the Northern Hemisphere. It is primarily a first-aid injury remedy when cold rather than warmth soon brings welcome, soothing relief.

**n o t e s** • Puncture wounds from nails or splinters, bites and stings, when pain is eased by cold compresses. • Wounds that look puffy and feel cold. • Injuries to the eye which looks cold, puffy and bloodshot.

# LYCOPODIUM
Lycopodium clavatum

This remedy is prepared from the spores of club moss, a strange prostrate plant which likes to grow on heaths. It is generally prescribed constitutionally for aiding chronic conditions but it can also be very helpful for digestive problems and sometimes even acute sore throats.

**n o t e s** • Conditions which are worse on the right side, or move from the right to the left side of the body.
• Flatulence and pain in the abdomen or stomach. • Problem is aggravated by gassy foods such as beans.

# CANTHARIS
Lytta vesicatoria

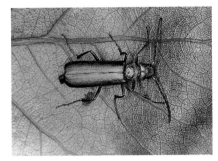

Cantharis is one of a few homeopathic remedies prepared from insects. It is derived from an iridescent green beetle which is commonly called Spanish fly. It is also known as the blister beetle because it is actually a major irritant if handled. It has an affinity with the urinary tract.

**n o t e s** • Cystitis – where there are highly uncomfortable, intense, burning-pains on urinating. • Evidence of burns or burning pains generally, as you would normally expect to get following sunburn, or burns from a hot pan.

# MAG PHOS
Magnesia phosphorica

Magnesia phosphorica is one of the 12 tissue salts, as well as being a proven remedy. It is well known that it works directly in helping to ease tension in the nerves as well as in the muscles. It can therefore be considered as a very effective painkiller.

**n o t e s** • Violent, cramping and spasmodic pains, often in the abdominal area. • Pains better for warmth, gentle massage and doubling up.
• Can help with colic, period pains, sciatica, toothache and earache.

# CHAMOMILLA
Matricaria chamomilla

Chamomile is a member of the daisy family. It strongly affects the nervous system. It is one of the most important medicines for the treatment of children: Aconite, Belladonna and Chamomilla are together known as the "ABC" remedies.

**n o t e s** • Bad temper and irritability.
• Teething problems in angry babies.
• In cases of colic, the stools are usually offensive, slimy and green.
• Extreme sensitivity to pain.
• The child's temper is considerably improved on being rocked or carried.

# MERCURIUS
Mercurius solubilis

The name of this remedy is sometimes abbreviated to Merc sol. It is prepared from the liquid metal mercury. It is used in acute septic states (infected areas) where the glands and their secretions are particularly affected.

**n o t e s** • Swollen and tender glands.
• Profuse sweating and increased thirst. • Breath, sweat and secretions can be offensive. • The tongue looks flabby, yellow and coated.
• Fevers blow hot and cold.
• Irritability and restlessness.

# PHOSPHORUS
Phosphorus

Phosphorus is an important constituent of the body, particularly of the bones. It can be useful in acute situations. These include digestive problems, with immediate vomiting once the food is warmed in the stomach, and constant diarrhoea. Phosphorus can also help aid minor haemorrhages (i.e. nosebleeds). It also relieves the "spacey" feeling that lingers too long after an anaesthetic.

**n o t e s** • Suits people who are lively, open and friendly, but who are also occasionally nervous and anxious.

## PHYTOLACCA
Phytolacca decandra

Phytolacca or poke-root is a well-known erect, unpleasant smelling plant that grows across the Northern Hemisphere, and also in South America. It is a glandular remedy that particularly affects the tonsils, and also the mammary glands. It is reckoned that Phytolacca is probably the most important remedy for helping in the treatment of mastitis.

**n o t e s** • Sore throats that look dark and angry. • Sore throats in which the pain feels like a hot ball. • Swollen, tender breasts with cracked nipples.

## PULSATILLA
Pulsatilla nigricans

Pulsatilla is one of the most useful of acute remedies, as well as being a very important constitutional one. The remedy comes from the pasque flower and is also known as the weathercock remedy because it suits people whose moods and symptoms are constantly changing. For this reason, it is considered a wonderful remedy for small children.

**n o t e s** • Tendency to be weepy and clingy. • Suits people with gentle, sympathetic natures.• Yellow-green discharge from the eyes or nose.

## RHUS TOX
Rhus toxicodendron

The remedy is prepared from poison ivy, native to North America. Its main use is in sprains, strains and swollen joints, but because of its itchy, rashy picture it can be a good remedy for illnesses such as chickenpox or shingles. It is also a useful remedy for acute rheumatism.

**n o t e s** • Extreme restlessness with a red, itchy rash. • Stiffness in the joints, which is eased by gentle motion. • The symptoms are far better for warmth, and considerably worse with cold, damp and over-exertion.

## RUTA
Ruta graveolens

Ruta, or rue, is a much valued, highly attractive garden plant with blue-green leaves. It is also an ancient herbal remedy that has been often called the herb of grace. It acts particularly well on the joints, tendons, cartilages and periosteum (the membrane that covers the bones). It also has an affinity with the eyes.

**n o t e s** • Bruises to the bones. • Strains to the joints and connecting tissue, especially to the ankles and wrists. • The symptoms are worse for cold and damp and better for warmth.

## SEPIA
Sepia officinalis

Sepia is a remedy prepared from the ink of the squid or cuttlefish. Normally its use should be left to the professional homeopath as it has a "big" picture (i.e. it can be used in many circumstances), but because of its affinity with the female reproductive system it can be helpful in some menstrual problems.

**n o t e s** • Suits tired, depressed, emotionally withdrawn people. • Morning sickness in pregnancy, which is worse for the smell of food. • Hot flushes during the menopause.

## SILICA
Silicea

Silica is a mineral derived from flint. It is one of the 12 tissue salts, and its presence in the body aids the vital elimination of toxins. It can be used acutely in septic (infected) conditions to strengthen the body's resistance to continual infection, and also to help expel any foreign bodies such as splinters.

**n o t e s** • Suitable for symptoms that are slow to heal, or for people who feel the cold, or who lack stamina or vitality. • Small-scale infections that seem to be turning septic rather than healing.

## SPONGIA
Spongia tosta

Spongia, as its name clearly indicates, is a remedy which is prepared from the lightly roasted skeleton part of the marine sponge. It actually works very well on the respiratory tract, and it is now generally considered to be one of homeopathy's major cough remedies. It is actually a significant and indeed important aid or remedy when it comes to treating croup in young children.

**n o t e s** • Dry spasmodic cough.
• The cough sounds like a saw being pulled through wood.

## NUX VOMICA
Strychnos nux vomica

Nux vomica is prepared from the seeds of the poison nut tree of South-east Asia. It is a remedy that has many uses in both chronic and acute situations, and it is known to be very useful when the digestive system is involved.

**n o t e s** • Nausea or vomiting after a rich meal, when the food remains undigested like a load in the stomach.
• A feeling that if only you could vomit you would feel better. • An urge to pass a stool, but with unsatisfactory results. • Heartburn.

## SYMPHYTUM
Symphytum officinale

The remedy is easily prepared from the common herb comfrey. It is also called knitbone, which indicates its main use in promoting the healing of broken bones. Use the remedy daily for several weeks after the bone has been set. Symphytum can also be used for many injuries to the eyeball such as, for example, getting a tennis ball directly in the eye.

**n o t e s** • Speeds up the knitting or fusing together of broken bones.
• Injuries to the eyeball, such as being hit by a hard object.

## VALERIAN
Valeriana officinalis

Valerian is a well-known herb whose overuse in the 19th century caused insomnia and over-taxation of the nervous system to the point of hysteria. Because of the principle "like cures like", very tiny doses such as those used in homeopathy can cure these very same problems. Valerian is an important remedy for sleeplessness. Take one pill about one hour before bedtime. You should soon notice the improvement.

**n o t e s** • Especially useful when the mind feels like a "hamster on a wheel".

## VERBASCUM
Verbascum thapsus

Verbascum is prepared from the great mullein, a common wayside herb. It is a highly regarded garden plant sending up marvellous stems. Homeopathically it is associated with earaches, and it is best used as an oil. The remedy is especially helpful for children, who tend to suffer from ear infections more often than adults. Place a few drops of the oil on a warmed teaspoon and gently insert into the ear, with the child lying on one side.

**n o t e s** • Earaches of all kinds, both in children and adults.

## VIBURNUM OPULUS
Viburnum opulus

The guelder rose is widely distributed in woods and damp places throughout northern Europe and the US. It is a valued garden plant, especially in the form 'Roseum' which has large white flowers, giving rise to its common name, the snowball tree. It is also known as cramp bark and the homeopathic remedy, which is prepared from the bark, can be very helpful for period pains as well as for spasmodic cramps.

**n o t e s** • For aiding the treatment of severe cramping and muscle spasms.

ayurveda
ayurveda

# ayurveda

Ayurveda is acknowledged as the traditional healing system of India. Thousands of years old, it has influenced many other healing systems around the world. In fact, it was already established before the births of Buddha and Christ, and some biblical stories clearly reflect the wisdom of the ancient Ayurvedic teachings.

There are many different branches to Ayurveda because it covers so many aspects of health and healing. They have been touched upon in the following pages, but the main emphasis is on diet and lifestyle, specifically tailored to the modern life.

Ayurvedic medicine is founded on the belief that all diseases stem from the digestive system and are caused either by poor digestion of food, which is the body's major source of nourishment, or by following an improper diet for your dosha (nature). Here you will find basic advice about suitable diets, as well as information about supportive treatments, including massage, exercise, colour, crystals, herbs and spices. There is also a list of common ailments that can be treated.

The following basic Ayurvedic approach will help you to develop some simple ways to keep yourself balanced in these days of increasing worry and stress. Identify your dosha, learn how to live in accordance with your own true nature, and discover how you can at last begin to heal your vikruti (current emotional, physical or mental health conditions) with the use of the best basic Ayurvedic methods.

# what is ayurveda? It may be little known – and remarkably few

people seem to have heard of it – but Ayurveda is a highly respected, highly revered ancient

form of learning which has an amazing amount to teach us. It brings peace of body and mind,

important ways of seeing the world and your own place in the scheme of things, and highly

practical, sensible ideas when it comes to medicine, diet and ways of staying calm and relaxed.

## THE ORIGINS OF AYURVEDA

The origins of Ayurveda are uncertain. It is recounted that thousands of years ago, men of wisdom or rishis (meaning seers) as they are known in India, were saddened by the suffering of humanity. They knew that ill health and short lives allowed man little time to consider his spirituality and to commune with the divine – with God.

In the Himalayan mountains they prayed hard and meditated together, calling upon God to help them to relieve the plight of man, and God felt moved by compassion and gave them the essential teachings that would enlighten them in the ways of healing illness, and thereby alleviate and remove all suffering on the earth.

It is believed that these teachings are the Vedas, although this cannot be proven, due to the lack of historical records. A book called the *Atharva Veda* was one of the first detailed accounts of the system. From this, and perhaps other ancient writings, came

*Indian sadhus, like the one shown here, tend to live a nomadic life, renouncing worldly goods, and devoting themselves to prayer.*

the beginnings of Ayurvedic medicine, which has developed, changed and absorbed many other influences over hundreds of years to become what it is today. Due to the invasions of India over the years, and the subsequent suppression of many original Indian ways of life, several ancient texts have been lost or even destroyed, but enough have survived to ensure the active continuation of these highly valued, greatly respected teachings.

Ayurveda is now acknowledged as the traditional healing system of India. It comes from two Sanskrit words, *ayur*, meaning "life", and *veda*, meaning "knowing", and can be interpreted as meaning the "science of life". The oldest healing system to remain intact, it is very comprehensive and has influenced many healing systems around the world.

*Ayurveda travelled out of India and influenced many other countries with its ageless wisdom about living in the light of truth.*

*The influence of Ayurveda has spread far and wide. This is reflected in the different oils that are used. Many are made from plants that are found all over the world, not just India.*

## THE INFLUENCE OF AYURVEDA

For centuries after the end of the Vedic era, Ayurvedic medicine developed into a comprehensive healing system. Its philosophy and techniques soon spread far and wide to China, Arabia, Persia and Greece, gradually influencing Middle Eastern, Greek and Chinese methods of healing. It is well known that Ayurvedic practitioners reached the ancient city of Athens, and it can be noted that the traditional Greek folk medicine, based upon the bodily humours (characteristics), is significantly similar to Ayurveda. In turn, Greek medicine strongly influenced the subsequent development of what we call traditional or orthodox Western medicine. However, it is much too difficult to say exactly how much or to what degree the medical philosophy of Ayurveda was indeed influential, or even how much Ayurveda influenced current techniques.

### Greek and European Medicine

The five elements in Chinese medicine appear to have come from Ayurveda. It is documented that the Indian medical system was brought to China by Indian Buddhist missionaries, many of whom were skilled Ayurvedic practitioners. The missionaries also travelled to South east Asia and Tibet, influencing the people of these lands. Tibetan medicine, for example, is an intricate mix of Ayurvedic practices and philosophy with a Tibetan Buddhist and shamanic influence.

## WHAT IS AYURVEDIC MEDICINE?

The main aim of Ayurvedic medicine (which is only one branch of Ayurveda) is to improve health and longevity, leaving the individual free to contemplate matters of the spirit and to follow a spiritual path. This does not mean that you have to be spiritual or religious to benefit from Ayurvedic medicine; the system is very practical in its applications and deals with all kinds of health problems, without spirituality ever being mentioned. Its main focus is nutrition, supported primarily by the use of herbs, massage and aromatic oils, but there are many complementary branches as well.

Ayurvedic philosophy encourages those who practise it to eat the fruits and seeds of the earth, rather than take the life of animals. Since some animal products have in fact been included in this introductory guide, they should only ever be used in strict moderation. Let common sense and sensitivity be your guide.

The branches of Ayurvedic medicine include specific diets, surgery, jyotish (Vedic astrology), psychiatry and pancha karma (cleansing and detoxifying techniques). Yoga is not a branch of Ayurveda, but since it shares the same roots you will find that the two are often practised together. Yoga includes meditation, mantras (prayer chants), yantras (contemplation of geometric visual patterns) and hatha yoga (practices for bringing great harmony to the spirit, mind and body).

If you are actually much more interested in the many spiritual aspects of Ayurvedic teachings, then it is strongly recommended that you think very seriously about taking up yoga so that it becomes a regular part of your life.

*Most people clearly benefit from meditation or yoga, which can help to illuminate the pathway to inner relaxation and peace.*

# the doshas
Instead of using modern psychology to group people into types, try using the ancient doshas. They pinpoint and identify three basic types of people, which in turn helps you to a greater self-awareness and to an appreciation of others. The doshas are also excellent ways of helping you to fine-tune and regulate your lifestyle, bringing greater peace and well-being. The doshas are not just terms, they are ways of actively improving your life.

## THE SEASONS

There are three doshas (basic types of people, in terms of constitution) – vata, pitta and kapha. They are influenced by the rhythms of nature, seasonal change and the time of year. Autumn is a time of change when leaves turn brown and dry; vata is highest in the autumn and early winter, and at times of dry, cold and windy weather. Pitta is highest in late spring, throughout the summer and during times of heat and humidity. Kapha is highest in the winter months and during early spring, when the weather is frequently still cold and damp.

In Ayurvedic theory, the progress of a disease goes through several stages. There is accumulation (when it is increasing), followed by aggravation (when it is at its highest point and can cause problems). There is also decrease (when it is lessening) and a neutral time when it is passive (neither decreasing nor increasing). Use the questionnaire later in this chapter to discover your dosha, and see whether it is vata, pitta or kapha. People who are single types can refer to the dosha that scores the highest points on their questionnaire. Dual doshic types should vary their lifestyle to suit the seasonal changes, as shown in the dual doshas section.

*Yoga can be a very helpful way of balancing both the body and mind. After a few classes you are free to practise by yourself.*

## YOUR BODY TYPE

This section clearly outlines how you can identify your dosha or body type. Dosha means "that which tends to go out of balance easily." Your dosha is in fact your bio-type or prakruti ("nature"). You are made up of a mixture of the five elements – ether, wind, fire, water and earth, and will display certain recognizable characteristics depending on your personality and nature.

As well as your prakruti, you may also have a vikruti, which is your current state of mental or physical health. This develops throughout your life and may actually differ from your prakruti. It is important that you treat your vikruti first (how you are now), then go back to living with your prakruti. For example, you may have developed arthritis or back trouble over a long period, or you may be suffering from a cold or skin rash which lasts a few days. Once you have have cleared your condition, maintain your prakruti using a preventative treatment, such as diet, massage, oils, colours and scents.

*Levels of vata increase in the autumn when the weather is changeable. Surrounding yourself with flowers helps you relax.*

### Warming up/spring

*pitta accumulating, kapha aggravated, vata neutral*

### Hot/summer

*vata accumulating, pitta aggravated, kapha decreasing*

### Cooling/autumn

*vata aggravated, pitta decreasing, kapha neutral*

### Cold/winter

*vata decreasing, pitta neutral, kapha accumulating*

Apart from the three single doshas, there are four combinations, making a total of seven differing constitutional types: vata, pitta, kapha, vata/pitta (or pitta/vata), pitta/kapha (or kapha/pitta), kapha/vata (or vata/kapha), and vata/pitta/kapha. These may be either out of balance or in a state of balance.

To discover your prakruti and vikruti, answer the questionnaire twice. Also ask other people who know you well to fill out the questionnaire for you, to give you as clear a picture of yourself as possible. The first time you fill out the questionnaire, you should concentrate upon your current condition – your vikruti – recording your answers based upon your present and recent health history.

You can discover your prakruti by answering the questionnaire a second time, this time with answers based upon your entire lifetime. Fill out the questionnaire with your complete history in mind. This will give you a better idea about the difference between your vikruti and your prakruti. Once the answers to the questionnaire have revealed both your vikruti and your prakruti (they may be the same, which is fine), the information here can be used to treat both. Follow whichever dosha scores most highly (vata, pitta or kapha).

## ELEMENTAL ENERGIES

The elements are very important in Ayurveda. They descend from space (ether), down to air. Air descends into the fire element. Fire falls into the water element and water to earth, so that we move from the most rarefied elements (ether), to the most dense (earth). With this in mind, you will notice that the chart below follows a descending pattern of ether and air (vata), fire and water (pitta) and water and earth (kapha). Vata is a mixture of ether and air and is often translated as "wind". In the creation story of Ayurveda, vata leads the other doshas, because its combination of air and ether is actually the most rarefied. The elements move from the most refined down to the most dense. Consequently, if a vata is out of balance, the end result will be that the others will be out of balance as well.

Your age and the season of the year will also have an influence upon your doshic type. From childhood up to the teenage years you are influenced by kapha; from your teens to the age of 50 or 60 you tend to come under the pitta influence, and from 50 to 60 onwards you enter the vata phase of life.

Each dosha has a particular energetic principle which influences responses within the body. Everyone has all three doshas to an extent, but it is the ratio between each that is important, and that creates your individuality. Each dosha plays an important role in this equation and balancing act. For example, movement (vata) without the stability of kapha would simply end up in chaos, and the inactivity of kapha without activity and movement would quickly result in stagnation.

*A kapha type (water and earth) will be intuitive, sensitive and will dislike change but will be good at holding things together.*

| Element | Dosha | Cosmic link | Principle | Influence |
| --- | --- | --- | --- | --- |
| ether/air | vata | wind | change | activity/movement |
| fire/water | pitta | sun | conversion | metabolism/transformation |
| water/earth | kapha | moon | inertia | cohesion |

# You and Your Dosha

Working out exactly which dosha type you are is easily done, but before tackling the questionnaire on the opposite page, read the following notes very carefully. They put this huge wealth of information, and its references to skin types, lifestyle, and speech, into an objective framework, giving you a clearer perspective, helping you understand precisely what are called your humoral factors.

## WHICH TYPE ARE YOU?

The questionnaire opposite is designed to help you to assess your basic ratio of humoral factors. From this you can determine which diet, colours, exercise routines, crystals, oils and scents are most likely to suit you. By referring to the sections on which you score the most points, you will identify whether you are a vata, pitta or kapha dosha, or what is called a combination type. Read the questions and, to discover your prakruti, tick those descriptions which apply to you in general terms. Allocate two ticks to the statement that you think is most applicable to you; use one tick for a description that could also possibly apply, but if a particular description does not apply to you, then leave it unticked.

## Revealing your Vikruti

As has already been explained, your current condition, or vikruti, may not be the same as your underlying constitution, or prakruti. If you wish to discover whether or not this is the case, go through the questions a second time, this time using crosses instead of ticks. To reveal your vikruti, answer the questions according to how you have been feeling in the more recent past, and how the descriptions relate to your current health or condition, including any illnesses or other changes, no matter how subtle, that you are currently experiencing.

*Gems are used in Ayurveda only with a prescription from a jyotish (Vedic or Hindu astrologer), or from an Ayurvedic physician.*

When you are answering the questions, do make sure that you clearly focus either on your prakruti (your general state throughout life – ticks), or on your vikruti (current or recent state – crosses). To avoid any possible confusion, make sure that you finish with one set of answers before you start attempting to fill out and assess the questionnaire for a second time.

If you wish, you can answer the questionnaire a third time, separating questions about the mind from questions about the body. Use circles and squares to record your answers. This will indicate whether your body and mind are the same dosha. If they are different, follow the dietary advice for the mind. For example, if you have a kapha body and a pitta mind, follow the kapha eating and exercise plan, including the massage technique, and ensure that you have soothing colours and a calm environment.

## "Vata", "Pitta", and "Kapha"

Following the questionnaire are three sections headed "Vata", "Pitta" and "Kapha". Having discovered your vikruti (condition) or prakruti (constitution), turn to the pages relevant to your predominant dosha for detailed advice on reducing any excess

*Vatas need to learn how to be still because they tend to suffer from energy depletion, having the least amount of stamina.*

(vikruti), or to see how you can maintain your true character (prakruti). When referring to the various sections, do please read the information very carefully before you begin to put it into practice. Please also note that when using Ayurvedic medicinal herbs, you should take them only for as long as you are experiencing any obvious symptoms. You must check that the herbs are suited to your basic doshic needs; do this quite frequently, monitoring yourself even on a weekly basis.

When you begin to use any of the Ayurvedic prescriptions and techniques, do not be tempted to try and elaborate on them. This will do far more harm than good. The effect of the prescriptions lies in the ratio of the individual ingredients. Change this even in the subtlest way and all the good work may well be undone. Ayurveda is extremely complex and precise. For example, there are lengthy guidelines about the specific crystals that may be used to make a crystal infusion for each individual dosha. It is advisable that you do not make other infusions unless you are qualified or highly experienced; since crystals and gems can have a very powerful effect.

*Choose foods and herbs according to your doshic condition.*

### Discover your Dosha

Mark the questionnaire with either a √ (= your general constitution – prakruti) or x (= your current or recent state – vikruti).

| | **Vata** | **Pitta** | **Kapha** |
|---|---|---|---|
| HEIGHT | Very short, or tall and thin | Medium | Tall or short and sturdy |
| MUSCULATURE | Thin, prominent tendons | Medium/firm | Plentiful/solid |
| BODILY FRAME | Light, narrow | Medium frame | Large/broad |
| WEIGHT | Light, hard to gain | Medium weight | Heavy, gains easily |
| SWEAT | Minimal | Profuse, especially when hot | Moderate |
| SKIN | Dry, cold | Soft, warm | Moist, cool, possibly oily |
| COMPLEXION | Darkish | Fair, pink, red, freckles | Pale, white |
| HAIR AMOUNT | Average amount | Early thinning and greying | Plentiful |
| TYPE OF HAIR | Dry, thin, dark, coarse | Fine, soft, red, fair | Thick, lustrous, brown |
| SIZE OF EYES | Small, narrow or sunken | Average | Large, prominent |
| TYPE OF EYES | Dark brown or grey, dull | Blue/grey/hazel, intense | Blue, brown, attractive |
| TEETH AND GUMS | Protruding, receding gums | Yellowish, gums bleed | White teeth, strong gums |
| SIZE OF TEETH | Small or large, irregular | Average | Large |
| PHYSICAL ACTIVITY | Moves quickly, active | Moderate pace, average | Slow pace, steady |
| ENDURANCE | Low | Good | Very good |
| STRENGTH | Poor | Good | Very good |
| TEMPERATURE | Dislikes cold, likes warmth | Likes coolness | Aversion to cool and damp |
| STOOLS | Tendency to constipation | Tendency to loose stools | Plentiful, slow elimination |
| LIFESTYLE | Variable, erratic | Busy, tends to achieve a lot | Steady, can skip meals |
| SLEEP | Light, interrupted, fitful | Sound, short | Deep, likes plenty |
| EMOTIONAL TENDENCY | Fearful, anxious, insecure | Fiery, angry, judgemental | Greedy, possessive |
| MENTAL ACTIVITY | Restless, lots of ideas | Sharp, precise, logical | Calm, steady, stable |
| MEMORY | Good recent memory | Sharp, generally good | Good long term |
| REACTION TO STRESS | Excites very easily | Quick temper | Not easily irritated |
| WORK | Creative | Intellectual | Caring |
| MOODS | Change quickly | Change slowly | Generally steady |
| SPEECH | Fast | Clear, sharp, precise | Deep, slow |
| RESTING PULSE | | | |
| WOMEN | Above 80 | 70–80 | Below 70 |
| MEN | Above 70 | 60–70 | Below 60 |
| **Totals:** *Please add up* | **Vata** | **Pitta** | **Kapha** |

# vata

Vata types are known to be rather restless, cool people, who certainly notice the cold. When you have excess levels of vata, fear, depression and nervousness become quite marked, significant traits, and with repressed emotions comes a definite weakening of the immune system. However, by adopting the appropriate lifestyle, and making one or two changes, you will create a better balance within yourself, and find that you achieve much more.

The vata body type is usually thin and narrow. Vatas do not gain weight easily and are often restless by nature, especially when they are busy and active. They have dry hair and cool skin and a tendency to feel the cold. Their levels of energy are erratic, and they have to be very careful not to exhaust themselves, leading to inconsistency. They may find it quite hard to relax, which can lead to an overactive mind and insomnia.

Vata symptoms will be changeable, being cold by nature and therefore worse in cold weather. Any pain will worsen during change. Vata people can suffer from wind, low back pain, arthritis and nerve disorders. Vata types, because of their individual restless nature, certainly require a regular intake of nourishment, and they should sit down to eat or drink at regular times. Careful exercise should always be taken in moderation, clearly maintaining a gentle, regular, well-worked out routine that will help to keep the mind focused, and in perfect harmony with the body.

*Vata people should try to eat warming foods which are earthy and sweet, with the emphasis upon cooked foods, such as a bowl of dhal, rather than salads.*

**Elements:** ether and air.
**Climate:** dry and cold.
**Principle:** movement.
**Emotions:** fearful, anxious, apprehensive, sensitive, timid, lacking confidence, slightly nervous, changeable.
**Systems most affected by excess vata:** the nervous system and also the colon.
**Symptoms of excess vata:** flatulence, back pain, problems with circulation, dry skin, outbreaks of arthritis, constipation, and nerve disorders.

*In summer the vata quickly begins to accumulate as the heat of the sun begins to dry everything out. The best way to stop your skin from drying out too, so keeping it gently moist, is to use a top quality natural cream.*

## DIETARY TIPS

Vata people must always be quite careful, but not to the point that cooking suddenly becomes something of a difficult problem. The easy-to-follow, basic guidelines are as follows.

You must avoid all kinds of fried foods, no matter how tempting, and you should eat at regular intervals. Irregular huge meals are to be avoided at all costs. To reduce any excess vata, then follow the vata diet and recommendations in your eating and living plan. Always attempt to avoid any foods and other items that are not listed, as far as is possible. If animal products are a part of your diet, they should be used strictly in moderation.

## HERBS AND SPICES

Almond essence, asafoetida (hing), basil leaves, bay leaves, cardamom pods, coriander (cilantro), fennel, fresh ginger, marjoram, mint, nutmeg, oregano, paprika, parsley, peppermint, spearmint, tarragon, thyme, turmeric and vanilla.

## GRAINS AND SEEDS

Oats (cooked), pumpkin seeds, quinoa, rice (this includes all kinds and varieties), sesame seeds, sprouted wheat bread, sunflower seeds and wheat.

## NUTS, MEAT & FISH

Almonds, brazil nuts, cashews, hazelnuts, macadamias, pecans, pine nuts, pistachios and walnuts. Beef, chicken, duck, eggs, sea fish, shrimps and turkey.

## VEGETABLES

Artichokes, asparagus, beetroot, carrots, courgettes (zucchini), cucumber, daikon radish, green beans, leeks, okra, olives, onions (cooked), parsnips, pumpkins, radishes, spinach (cooked), swede (rutabagas), sweet potatoes, tomatoes (cooked), and fresh watercress.

## FRUIT

Apricots, avocados, bananas, berries, cherries, fresh coconuts, dates, fresh figs, grapefruit, grapes, lemons, limes, mangoes, melons, oranges, peaches, pineapples, rhubarb and strawberries.

## DAIRY PRODUCTS

Cow's milk, cottage cheese, goat's milk, goat's' cheese and soft cheese – all are to be taken sensibly, in moderation.

## COOKING OILS

Unrefined sesame oil.

## DRINKS

Apricot juice, carrot juice, ginger tea, grape juice, grapefruit juice, orange juice, hot dairy drinks, lemon balm tea, lemonade and peach juice.

## AROMAS AND MASSAGE OILS

Vata people are unusual because they tend to benefit much more than either of the other two doshas from having a massage. Consequently they should consider massaging their feet, hands and head every morning, and have a regular massage at least once a week. The massage should become a regular, greatly appreciated part of your lifestyle.

Vata aromas are warm and sweet, and the most appropriate massage oil for the vata personality is gently warmed sesame oil. Bottles of sesame oil are widely available, and are generally of a high, well-perfumed standard. If that is impossible to obtain, any other oil (preferably virgin olive) will suffice. It can be perfumed by the addition of your favourite herb. Oil is good for vata types, and if your vata is seriously out of balance, increase the number of massages you have a week from one to as many as three. You will soon notice the enormous improvement.

When using essential oils, note they must be diluted. Do not put them directly on your skin or take them internally. In fact it is not advisable to use the same essential oil for more than two weeks; interchange your essential oils so that you do not create a toxic build-up, or overload of one fragrance. If you are pregnant or have a diagnosed medical condition, do not use any essential oil without consulting a qualified practitioner.

Warm, calming or earthy essential oils are the most suitable for vata. These include camphor (which can be an irritant, so do test yourself for sensitivity first), eucalyptus, ginger, sandalwood and jatamansi (a spikenard species from India).

### vata massage

**1** The correct vata massage should always be gentle.

**2** Keep the actions firm, regular, soothing and relaxing.

**3** Use flowing, continuous stroking movements.

**4** Oil and ease any areas displaying dry, tight skin.

## COLOURS

Vata individuals generally benefit from most of the pastel colours, and from earthy colours that are gentle and warm to look at. They include ochres, browns and yellows.

### Ochre

A warm, friendly and relaxing colour, ochre is good at drawing the energy down, right through the system, helping the vata individual to feel much more solid and steady.

### Brown

A solid, reliable colour, brown helps to ground the vata type, stabilizing any tendency to flightiness. It is also good at holding the emotions in place; it consolidates and aids concentration.

### Yellow

A warming, enlivening colour, yellow is linked to the mind and intellect. It helps to keep the vata mentality alert by focusing the mind, and calming any rising emotions.

### Making a Colour Infusion

Begin by taking a piece of thin cotton or silk. The fabric should be warm yellow in colour, and sufficiently thin to allow the light through. Next, wrap it around a small transparent (not coloured) jar filled with spring water and leave it outside in the sunlight for four hours. Finally, remove the fabric. Note, vata infusions should not be stored in the fridge, but kept at room temperature.

*This infusion will encourage a sense of warmth and well-being.*

## GEMS AND CRYSTALS

Gems and crystals have subtle healing qualities that can be utilized in Ayurvedic medicine. Their curious, well-known powers are taken seriously by the jyotish (Vedic astrologer), who can determine which gems or crystals you will need to use, depending on the circumstances of your life chart.

Topaz is a warm stone that traditionally dispels fear, making it an ideal stone for vata because it calms high emotions and anxiety. Wear topaz whenever you want to feel confident and in control. Amethyst is an appropriate crystal to wear when you want to balance vata. It soon promotes a fine clarity of mind and thought, and will help you to radiate harmony.

There may be times when it is advisable to remove all crystals – when you find circumstances in your life are changing for the worse. This indicates that your birth chart or constitution does not require the healing qualities of a particular crystal, or that it is highlighting an area of your birth chart in a negative way. Seek expert advice on replacements.

### Cleaning Crystals and Crystal Infusions

Before making a crystal infusion, it is best to cleanse your crystal. In fact, crystals that are used for infusions should ideally be cleansed before and after each use. Once you have filled a bowl with spring water, dissolve a teaspoon of sea salt in it. The crystal sits in for up to about eight hours before being rinsed.

**1** Place the crystal in the water and leave to stand for about four hours, or leave it overnight in the dark.

**2** Rinse it in spring water, visualizing any residues that were being held in the crystal being washed away.

To make a crystal infusion, take the cleansed crystal and hold it in your hands, imagining that the crystal is full of peace and calm. Place the crystal in a clear glass bowl, cover it with spring water, and leave it in the sunlight for about four hours. Remove the crystal and bottle the spring water. You can now drink the infusion prior to any mentally demanding tasks. It will aid clarity of mind and help reduce any stress that might arise as a result of pressure. You can keep the infusion for just 24 hours, after which it should be discarded. Make sure you store the infusion away from domestic appliances and electrical equipment.

## EXERCISE AND TONIC

Since vata is cold in nature it benefits from warmth and comfort. Make your own warming tonic drinks for cold windy days by combining ingredients from the vata eating plan. Be aware though that sugar weakens the immune system and vatas, with their tendency to stress (another immune suppressor), need to be particularly wary of sugary and refined foods, choosing naturally sweet-tasting foods, such as fruit, instead.

Vata people benefit from gentle, relaxing forms of exercise. Being the most easily exhausted of the various categories, they should be careful not to overdo things. Examples of suitable exercise include walking, yoga and slow swimming. In essence, it is not so much the form of exercise that you take, but rather the way in which you take it. With vata, the exercise routine should always be on the gentle side; with this in mind, vata types can undertake most sports and activities.

Yoga stretches will gradually and gently lengthen your muscles, and increase your flexibility. It has enormous all-round benefits. If you do not actively practise yoga as a form of exercise, you may well find that achieving a full or even half lotus for meditation is much too strenuous and difficult. If this is the case, do not try and force yourself. Instead, use a specifically designed meditation stool, or place some firm cushions on the floor beneath you. Push your bent knees on to the floor, then tuck your feet in towards you on the floor, forming a solid triangular base with your legs.

### Fresh Ginger and Lemon Tea

This tea is remarkably quick and easy to make, and tastes absolutely delicious. It is also a marvellous tonic for a vata.

*1 lemon*
*A small slice of fresh ginger*

*Spring water*
*Raw honey or fructose*

**1** Wash the lemon and then cut it into thin slices, leaving the peel on. Peel the piece of fresh ginger and slice it finely.
**2** Place the lemon and ginger slices in a small teapot.
**3** Add boiling spring water, then stir. Finally sweeten with honey or fructose, drink and enjoy.

# pitta

Pitta people are generally quite well-balanced, well-proportioned, rounded types, admired by all, but they can suddenly become passionately focused and intense. At its most extreme this tendency leads to a high degree of intolerance and irritability. Consequently pitta types should keep well away from any foods that are known to be hot and spicy, and which might inflame them, and concentrate on meals that promote their more soothing side.

The pitta body type is usually of average build and nicely proportioned. Pittas like food and have a healthy appetite. The hair is usually straight, fine and fair, though dark-haired people can also be pitta types. People with red hair will automatically have some level of pitta within their nature. Like the fire element, their temperament can be quite intense, and when it manifests itself in excess this can lead to marked intolerance.

Pitta skin will have a tendency to be sensitive to the sun, and pitta types will need to be very careful how much time they spend in direct sunlight. The fiery nature of the sun will sometimes inflame the pitta person, leading to skin rashes, freckles and sunburn. Cool showers, cool environments and plenty of long cooling drinks (but not ice-cold ones) will help to alleviate any high temperatures and calm down pitta types.

People of this nature can be impatient, having highly active and alert minds. However, pitta people can also have a very good sense of humour and a warm personality.

*Pitta people should always aim to eat food that is rather soothing. What they must do is avoid any foods that are considered hot and spicy. Ingredients such as fiery chillies are definitely off the menu.*

**Elements:** fire and water.
**Climate:** hot and moist.
**Principle:** transformation.
**Emotions:** hate, anger, resentment, intolerance, impatience, irritability, indignation, jealousy, good humour, intelligence, alertness, open warm-heartedness.
**Systems most affected by excess pitta:** skin, metabolism, small intestines, eyes, liver, hair on the head.
**Symptoms of excess pitta:** skin disorders, acidity, sun-sensitivity, premature degrees of hair loss or loss of hair colour, outbreaks of diarrhoea.

*Pitta types generally benefit from spending time away from fast, noisy, chaotic urban environments. They should seek out quiet, peaceful, well-shaded, naturally calming surroundings.*

## DIETARY TIPS

The pitta person should avoid all hot, spicy and sour foods, as they will aggravate this dosha; they should also avoid all fried foods. Since heated food will increase pitta within the system, pitta types should eat more raw than cooked foods. As a primarily vegetarian system, Ayurveda does not advocate the eating of animal products, especially for the pitta dosha, so although some meats and other animal products have been included in the following list, they should really be used in the strictest moderation. Let common sense always prevail.

## HERBS AND SPICES

Aloe vera juice (totally avoid during a pregnancy), basil leaves, cinnamon, coriander (cilantro), cumin, dill, fennel, fresh ginger, hijiki, mint leaves, spearmint.

## GRAINS AND SEEDS

Barley, basmati rice, flax seeds, psyllium seeds, rice cakes, sunflower seeds, wheat, wheat bran, white rice.

## PROTEINS

Aduki beans, black beans, black-eyed beans, chick peas (garbanzos), kidney beans, lentils (red and brown), lima beans, mung beans, pinto beans, soya beans, split peas, tempeh and tofu. Chicken, freshwater fish, rabbit, turkey.

## VEGETABLES

Artichokes, asparagus, broccoli, Brussels sprouts, butternut squash, cabbages, courgettes (zucchini), celery, cucumber, fennel, green beans and green peppers, Jerusalem artichokes, kale, leafy greens, leeks, lettuces, mushrooms, onions (cooked), parsnips, spinach (cooked). Eat most vegetables raw instead of cooked.

## FRUIT

Apples, apricots, avocados, berries, cherries, dates, figs, mangoes, melons, oranges, pears, pineapples, plums, pomegranates, prunes, quinces, raisins, red grapes and watermelons. Always make sure that the fruits have fully ripened, and are very sweet and fresh.

## DAIRY PRODUCTS

Cottage cheese, cow's milk, diluted yoghurt, ghee (clarified butter), goat's milk, mild soft cheeses and unsalted butter may all be taken but with a reasonable degree of moderation.

## COOKING OILS

Olive oil, sunflower oil, soya and walnut oil. As with all dairy products, these oils should be used in moderation.

## DRINKS

Apple juice, apricot juice, cool dairy drinks, grape juice, mango juice, mixed vegetable juice, soya milk, vegetable bouillon, elderflower tea, jasmine tea, spearmint tea and strawberry tea.

## AROMAS AND MASSAGE OILS

Essential oils for pitta include honeysuckle, jasmine, sandalwood and vetiver. They must be diluted and should never be taken internally. Avoid a toxic build-up by interchanging the oils every two weeks. If you are pregnant or have a diagnosed medical condition, you must consult a qualified practitioner before attempting to use essential oils.

If possible go to an experienced masseur. They understand exactly how a massage should be given. In time you will pick up the basics and may be able to start giving others a gentle massage. The key to success is to take your time, and make sure that your partner is fully relaxed. There is no point in attempting a soft massage when they are in an agitated state, and are incapable of lying still for a couple of minutes, let alone 20. When applying the essential oils, it is important that you work with firm, consistent hand movements, totally avoiding any sudden changes of direction. Think of your hands as waves, sweeping in one long curving movement over a smooth beach. That said, do not go to the opposite extreme and be so frightened of touching or hurting the skin that you barely make any contact. The right degree of pressure is about the same as for a firm hairwash.

After the massage, do not expect to get up and rush out. That would immediately undermine all the good work. Instead, take your time, possibly even have a cat-nap, and only step back into everyday life when you are feeling absolutely ready. That way you will feel refreshed, calm and clear-headed. It also helps if you have a massage on a day that you know will be stress-free.

## Pitta Massage

**1** Start the massage in the middle of the back.

**2** Use continuous, relaxing, deep, varied movements.

**3** Be gentle on any areas of stiffness or soreness.

**4** Continue with sweeping, slow movements.

## COLOURS

If you are experiencing symptoms of excess pitta, such as irritability or impatience, or on occasions when you know that you are going to have a busy and active day ahead of you, balance your system by wearing natural fibres in cooling and calming colours, such as green, blue, violet or any quiet pastel shade.

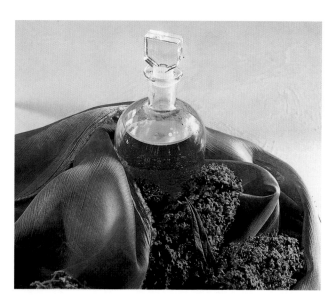

### Blue

Blue is a soothing, healing colour which is ideal for the active pitta type. It is linked to spiritual consciousness and helps the pitta to remain open and calm without being over-stimulated.

### Green

Green, an integral colour of the natural world, brings harmonious feelings to the pitta personality, having the ability to soothe emotions and calm passionate feelings.

### Violet

Violet is a refined colour that soothes and opens the mind, and increases awareness of spiritual issues.

### Making a Colour Infusion

Take a piece of thin, translucent cotton or silk in violet or light blue. Wrap it around a small transparent (not coloured) bottle or jar filled with spring water. Leave it outside in dappled sunlight, not in direct sun, for approximately six hours. Finally, remove the fabric, and drink the infusion to encourage the wonderful sensation of inner peace and harmony.

*A blue colour infusion will help to clear the system of a build-up of pressure.*

## GEMS AND CRYSTALS

When you want to reduce excess pitta, wear pearls or a mother-of-pearl ring set in silver upon the ring finger of your right hand. Pearls have the ability to reduce inflammatory conditions, including sudden passionate, heated emotions. Ideally, natural pearls should be worn, although cultured pearls are actually quite acceptable. The most harmonious day to put on your pearls is a Monday (the moon's day) during a new moon. However, do not wear pearls when you have a kapha condition, such as a cold. The moonstone has the ability to calm emotions and is soft and cooling, being feminine in orientation. It can certainly help to pacify the pitta personality.

You can also use stones, as shown right, to make a special infusion. It involves no more than placing the stone in a glass bowl that has been topped up with spring water. The key part of the process is standing the bowl and stone outside, preferably on a night when there is a full moon and a cloudless sky. The longer you can leave it standing out the better, three hours being about the minimum period for successful results.

When you bring in the bowl, pour the special water into a clean glass and drink before breakfast. If you can make standing this bowl outside at night a regular part of your routine, then you will soon notice the difference that drinking moonstone water makes. You will feel increasingly calm, relaxed, clear-headed, stable, grounded, and above all inwardly strong. Your confidence grows and grows. You will find that other people definitely notice, and become increasingly attracted towards you. Feeling more attractive actually gives you a new lease of life.

## Making a Moonstone Infusion

**1** Take a stone specimen that has already been cleansed.

**2** Leave the bowl outside to stand under a full moon.

**3** Remove the moonstone, and pour out the liquid.

**4** Drink the moonstone infusion when you wake.

---

### Orange and Elderflower Infusion

This infusion makes a light refreshing drink, ideal in summer.

| | |
|---|---|
| *1 large sweet orange* | *300ml/½ pint spring water* |
| *2 heads fresh elderflower* | *Fructose to taste* |
| *Fresh spearmint* | |

**1** Wash the orange in spring water. Slice and put in a jug.
**2** Add elderflower heads and spearmint; pour in spring water.
**3** Leave for one hour, add fructose to taste, and drink.

## EXERCISE AND TONIC

Cooling drinks made from fresh fruit and vegetable juices are ideal tonics for the pitta constitution.

Pittas require a moderate amount of exercise, which should involve some element of vigour and challenge – jogging, team sports and some of the gentler martial arts which do not stress sudden, fierce, aggressive movements. Pitta exercise should not overstimulate the body, and any exercise should be kept in line with an average amount of effort and challenge. You should avoid going to such extremes that your pitta nature gets carried away and you end up overdoing it. So, for example, doubles tennis is much better for you than singles, swimming is better than squash, and gentle jogging is much better for you than sudden sprinting. In the end, though, it is not so much what you do but how you do it that is deemed important.

This orange and elderflower infusion, left, is a light and delicate alternative to a cordial. Cordials are made by boiling all the ingredients together, which is not appropriate for pitta types because of the heat required in the cooking process. In fact, a general awareness of such techniques will help you make the right decisions in all aspects of your diet. Note that drinks are just as important as anything else you might have. They contribute greatly to our overall wellbeing.

# kapha

Kapha types are restless, complex, interesting contradictions. You will also find that despite being quite athletic, they actually need plenty of motivation, without which they can easily become overweight. On the plus side, they are certainly highly sensitive, but in return they do need quite a lot of sensitive handling. All in all they are thoroughly reliable, methodical people, and with that extra energy input will always stay one step ahead.

The kapha body type is well built, with a tendency to weight problems, especially if an exercise programme is not followed to keep the kapha active and moving. Kapha people are naturally athletic but they do need motivation. They are generally very sensitive and emotional, and they do require understanding otherwise they tend to turn to food as an emotional support and stabilizer. They should always ensure that what they eat is suitable for their body type. Their hair will be thick, fine and wavy, their skin soft, smooth and sensuous, and their eyes large, trusting and attractive.

Kapha people are inclined to be slow and steady, methodical and pragmatic, with a real dislike of change. They make good managers though, because they like to be reliable and available. They act like an anchor in a business because they have an innate organizing ability. Note that bright, strong, striking colours will greatly help to reduce any excess kapha, and stimulate those who are feeling slow, sluggish and dull.

*Kapha food should be light, dry, hot and stimulating. Always opt for cooked foods, such as hot and spicy vegetable curries, in preference to any kind of fresh salad.*

**Elements:** water and earth.
**Climate:** cold and damp.
**Principle:** cohesion.
**Emotions:** stubbornness, greed, jealousy, possessiveness, lethargy, reliability and methodical behaviour, kindliness, motherliness.
**Systems most affected by excess kapha:** joints, lymphatics, body fluids and mucous membranes throughout the body.
**Symptoms of excess kapha:** congestion, bronchial/nasal discharge, sluggish digestion, nausea, slow mental responses, idleness, desire for sleep, excess weight, fluid retention.

*Because kapha individuals have a tendency towards inertia, they need plenty of motivation. A good kick-start to the day is regular, early morning outdoor exercise, such as a brisk walk or a jog.*

## DIETARY TIPS

Kapha people should focus upon cooked food, but can have some salads occasionally. They should avoid fats and oils unless they are hot and spicy. Dairy products, sweet, sour and salty tastes and a high intake of wheat will also aggravate kapha. Although some meats and animal products have been included, they should always be used in moderation.

To reduce any excess levels of kapha (vikruti), or to maintain the right balance because you are a kapha dosha (prakruti), include the following items in your eating plan and try to avoid any foods that are not listed here.

## HERBS AND SPICES

Asafoetida (hing), black or Indian pepper, chilli pepper, coriander leaves (cilantro), dry ginger, garlic, horseradish, mint leaves, mustard, parsley or any other hot spices.

## GRAINS AND SEEDS

Barley, buckwheat, corn, couscous, oat bran, polenta, popcorn (plain), rye, sprouted wheat bread, toasted pumpkin seeds and occasional small quantities of toasted sunflower seeds.

## BEANS AND PULSES

Aduki beans, black-eyed beans, chick peas (garbanzos), lima beans, pinto beans, red lentils, split peas and tempeh.

## MEAT AND FISH

Eggs, freshwater fish, turkey, rabbit, shrimps and venison.

## VEGETABLES

Artichokes, broccoli, Brussels sprouts, cabbage, carrots, cauliflower, celery, daikon radish, fennel, green beans, kale, leeks, lettuce, mushrooms, okra, onions, peas, peppers, radishes, spinach. Kapha vegetables should be cooked.

## FRUITS

Apples, apricots, berries, cherries, peaches, pears, pomegranates and prunes.

## COOKING OILS

Corn, almond or sunflower oil may be used in small quantities.

## DRINKS

Fruit drinks should not contain sugar or additives. Recommended hot drinks include black tea, carrot juice, cranberry juice, grape juice, mango juice, mixed vegetable juice, nettle tea, passion flower tea, raspberry tea and occasional wine.

## AROMAS AND MASSAGE OILS

Kapha individuals require minimal oil or none at all with massage, using instead a natural, unscented talcum powder which can be purchased from most health food stores. If an essential oil is used at all, the best ones for kapha individuals include eucalyptus, cinnamon, orange peel (since this can cause sun sensitivity, avoid strong sunlight after a massage with orange peel), ginger and myrrh. All of these oils are stimulating and it would be well advisable, after diluting approximately 7–10 drops of essential oil in 25ml/1 fl oz carrier oil, to test an area of skin first to check for any possible sensitive reaction.

Unlike the sensitive gentleness of the pitta massage with its sweeping regular movements designed to relax, the kapha is actually quite fast and vigorous. You will notice that when having a massage the hands sweep over you firmly and energetically, keeping to a constant rhythm. If giving such a massage to a friend or partner, be aware that it can surprisingly be quite tiring. The aim is to kick-start and stimulate the metabolism that tends towards the sluggish.

Concentrate on the hip and groin areas to encourage lymphatic drainage, and also around the armpits to release any congestion. Finally, note as always that essential oils must be diluted and should not be taken internally. Do not to use the same essential oil for more than two weeks. If you are pregnant or have a diagnosed medical condition, do not use any essential oil without consulting a qualified practitioner. The risks are not worth taking.

## Kapha Massage

**1** Kapha massage needs to fairly vigorous and stimulating.

**2** Use fast movements, using talcum powder.

**3** Use hip/groin massage to assist lymphatic drainage.

**4** Another major lymph gland area is around the armpits.

---

## COLOURS

Kapha individuals benefit from the warm and stimulating colours of the spectrum. Whenever you experience symptoms such as lethargy and sluggishness, which suggest excess kapha, or if you need to be particularly active, wear bright, invigorating, stimulating colours. You will quickly notice how effective they are, inspiring a change in your temperament.

### Red

Red is the colour of blood and will increase circulation as well as being energizing and positive. It should be used sparingly to avoid over-stimulation of kapha, creating excess pitta.

### Orange

Orange is a warming, nourishing colour which feeds the sexual organs, and its glowing colour helps to remove congestion.

### Pink

Warm, comforting pinks gently stimulate kapha into activity. Being a softer colour than red, pink may be worn without ill-effects for significantly longer periods. A highly useful colour.

### Making a Colour Infusion

Take a piece of thin cotton or silk. The fabric should be a warm pink and sufficiently translucent to allow the light to penetrate. Wrap it around a transparent (not coloured) small bottle containing spring water. Stand it in full sunlight or upon a windowsill with the window open so that the light can fall naturally upon the bottle. Leave it for about four hours. Remove the fabric and drink the contents of the bottle within 24 hours.

*If possible, choose a fabric which has been dyed with natural dyes.*

## GEMS AND CRYSTALS

Lapis lazuli is a reliably suitable, highly useful crystal with which to reduce any excess levels of kapha. Known as the heavenly stone it will quickly help kapha individuals to increase their bodily vibrations, raising them from the level of the dense and slow to a much more refined and spiritual resonance. Lapis lazuli is a quite remarkable crystal, one that is well worth seeking out.

## Crystal Infusion

Cleanse your lapis lazuli prior to making an infusion. Hold the lapis in your hands for a few moments, visualizing clarity and inspiration. Take your time to get this right. The crystal should now be ready for use. Place it in a clear glass bowl and cover it with spring water. Leave it outside in the sunlight for about four hours. The brighter and sunnier the sky, the better. Next, remove the crystal, and bottle the infused spring water. You can regularly drink small amounts of it throughout the day, as required, and this will certainly ensure a continued rising of your spirits towards inspired, enlivened action.

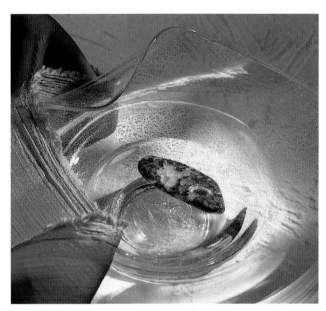

*Make a lapis infusion to reduce excess kapha.*

## EXERCISE AND TONIC

Kapha types may well avoid this page because it suggests exercise! However, kapha people must address their natural aversion to physical activity. Exercise will make an amazing difference, cleansing excess kapha, and making valuable room for their inner beauty and radiance to shine right through.

Since kapha individuals will tend to shy away from any vigorous exercise, a certain amount of self-discipline is required. Once a regular exercise routine is established, however, the kapha type will enjoy and benefit from the enlivened and energetic feeling that all activity and exercise brings. Examples of fairly vigorous exercise well suited to the kapha type include running, fast swimming, aerobics and even fitness training. If at all unused to such exercise, start with a gentle routine, and seek guidance from an expert, qualified trainer.

It is advisable to increase the exercise level during colder spells of weather when extra stimulation is required. If this becomes a regular routine it will really push the kapha type. The benefits will soon be obvious.

*Kapha people need to ensure that they have vigorous exercise, such as aerobics.*

### Spiced Yogi Tea

Spiced yogi tea is a delicious, warming drink which will soon help to reduce any excess kapha and is perfect for warming up cold bones on a chilly winter's day.

2.5ml/½ tsp dry ginger
4 whole cardamom pods
5 cloves
A pinch of black pepper or pippali (Indian long pepper)

1 large cinnamon stick
600ml/1 pint/2½ cups spring water
30ml/2tbsp goat's milk or organic soya milk

**1** Mix the spices together in a saucepan.
**2** Add the spring water and boil off half the liquid.
**3** Turn off the heat and add the goat's milk or soya milk.
**4** Stir and strain the liquid. Serve hot.

# dual doshas

In all relationships, at home and work, it will make a great difference if you can try to adopt the approaches recommended for your own particular dosha. The vata dosha may well need to work at being much more reliably consistent, with the pitta dosha aiming at far greater tolerance and patience. The rather possessive kapha dosha, on the other hand, should always put extra trust and flexibility right at the top of the list.

### Vata/Pitta – Pitta/Vata

If, when you answered the questionnaire in the introduction, you found that you scored twice as many points on any one type as on the other two, this means that you will predominantly be that type. For example, a score of 30 points on kapha and 5 or 10 on the others would indicate that you are a kapha type. However, if there is a closer gap with perhaps 30 points for kapha and 20 for pitta then you are classified as a kapha/pitta type. If you are such a dual type, read the following essential information.

Vata/pitta is a combination of ether/air and fire/water elements. If you belong to this dual type, refer to both the vata and the pitta eating and living plans. Choose items from the pitta plan during the spring and summer months, and during outbreaks of hot, humid weather. Follow the vata plan during the autumn and winter months, and during any cold, dry spells. For example, pungent foods aggravate pitta but can actually help to calm vata (because vata is cold), which is why the plans need to be changed in accordance with the weather, your health and a wide range of other factors. It is really quite important that you keep

*Vata/pitta – pitta/vata herbs include the different kinds of basil, coriander (cilantro), cumin seeds, fennel, mint, turmeric and vanilla pods.*

a regular, accurate check on such factors, and modify your approach accordingly.

Eat your vegetables in season, and mostly cooked and flavoured with appropriate vata spices to minimize aggravation of vata and pitta. Only small amounts of bitter vegetables should be used. Among foods suitable for the vata/pitta type are broccoli, cauliflower, cucumber, endive, kale, onion (cooked), plantain, coconut, sweet oranges, apricots and other sweet fruits. Teas that are beneficial include elderflower, fennel, lemon balm and rosehip teas. Appropriate herbs and spices for vata/pitta – pitta/vata include fresh basil, caraway, cardamom, cumin, fennel, garam masala, spearmint and vanilla.

The nature of vata is change and when you are more familiar with the doshic influences that the climate has on you, you may be more flexible with the doshic recommendations. Remember, though, that you are influenced by everything touching your life.

*Your lifestyle can be affected by your health. Pitta or vata doshas should find time to create a calming and restful ambience in which to relax and wind down.*

*If you belong to the vata/pitta type, eat plenty of sweet, ripe fruits, such as melons and oranges, when they are in season.*

## Pitta/Kapha – Kapha/Pitta

This is a combination of the fire, water and earth elements. If you belong to this dual type, follow the kapha eating and living plan during the winter months and during spells of cold, damp weather, and take note of the pitta plan during the summer months, and during hot, humid weather.

You should always choose foods that are pungent and astringent, such as onions, celery, lemons, dandelion, mustard greens and watercress, and eat fresh fruit and vegetables. All fruit juices should be diluted with water or milk. Suitable teas for the pitta/kapha – kapha/pitta type include bancha twig, blackberry, dandelion, jasmine, licorice (not to be used if you suffer from high blood pressure or oedema) and spearmint. The herbs, spices and flavourings that apply to the pitta/kapha type include coriander, dill leaves, fennel, kudzu, orange peel, parsley, rosewater, and sprigs of refreshing spearmint.

## Vata/Kapha – Kapha/Vata

Vata/kapha is a combination of ether, air, water and earth. You should follow the kapha eating and living plan during the winter and spring months, and during cold, damp weather. You should stick to the vata plan during the autumn and summer months, and during any cold, dry windy spells.

Since the vata/kapha type is cold, you should therefore be encouraged to have plenty of pungent, hot and spicy foods. Chinese and Eastern cuisine is a "must". Good examples of suitable foods include artichokes, asparagus, mustard greens, parsnips, summer and winter squashes and watercress. Vegetables with seeds should be well cooked with the appropriate vata spices to minimize any possible aggravation.

It is equally important to eat plenty of fresh seasonal fruits, and they include apricots, berries, cherries, lemons, mangoes, peaches and strawberries. The vata/kapha type should be very careful to avoid a mono-diet of brown rice.

The herbs and spices for this particular type include allspice, anise, asafoetida (hing), basil, black pepper, basil, cinnamon, coriander, cumin, curry powder, garlic, nutmeg, poppy seeds, saffron and vanilla.

## Tridosha

In very rare instances a person may score more or less equally for all three doshas, revealing themselves to be all three types, or what is known as "tridosha" (literally, three-doshas). If you are this interesting combination of three doshas you will require a specially formulated tridoshic diet and living plan. Since your make-up is more elaborate than for single types, your plan is accordingly more interesting and varied. The onus is on you, however, to closely follow the seasonal changes and modify the agenda as appropriate, making sensible, sensitive modifications. Being a tridosha involves quite a degree of self-discipline, and a clever ability to switch promptly between all three lifestyle plans.

Always eat according to the weather and to your personal circumstances. For example, on hot days, and during the spring and summer months, follow the pitta plan; on cold days and during the winter months, follow the kapha plan; and during the late summer and autumn, or on windy days or during spells of cold dry weather, follow the vata plan.

If you find that you fall into this highly unusual, remarkable category, it will certainly be worthwhile seeking out and consulting an Ayurvedic practitioner to find out more about what being a tridosha entails.

*Pitta/kapha – kapha/pitta foods include curry leaves or powder, garam masala, mint, orange peel oil and rosewater.*

ayurvedic treatments
ayurvedic treatments

# ayurvedic treatments

The entire basis and the whole concept of Ayurvedic treatment is dietary; put bluntly, diet is exactly what it all leads back to – the tried and tested use and combination of specific foods. Fortunately, several excellent, imaginative Ayurvedic cookbooks with a wide range of tasty recipes have been published, and they are definitely well worth tracking down, collecting and studying if you want to learn more about Ayurvedic nutrition. They will make a great difference at meal times.

The following pages have been divided into several sections with the express purpose of outlining the basic characteristics of each type. This includes a wealth of vital information which forms the backbone, the foundation, and the essential core of the Ayurvedic approach. It deals with all kinds of related emotions, and the treatment systems closely associated with and most pertinent to each dosha. It also describes and explains the many symptoms of excess, together with a huge wealth of detail about what you should and should not be eating, which colours you really ought to be wearing, the scents and oils you should be using, the herbs and spices most beneficial to you, and the tonic recipes for each type, whether vata, pitta, or kapha.

In addition, there are key massage techniques, for example showing you how to follow the direction of the colon when massaging the stomach with brahmi oil, and which gem and crystal you should be working with in order to help you to reduce any excess levels in your dosha(s), thereby making sure they have a balanced, healthy relationship.

To the novice some of these ideas might seem slightly daunting, especially if you come from a background in which traditional forms of Western medicine have a stranglehold, but once they and the language in which they are expressed become familiar, you will see that the principles are actually very simple; they spell out some highly relevant advice. All you then have to do is to follow the right plan, whether you are trying to reduce an excess, or wish to build up and maintain the right balance in your system.

Once you become familiar with the many excellent Ayurvedic treatments, you can become slightly more adventurous. There is absolutely no reason why you should not start making up your own tonic recipes for your own body type. This is easily done by combining ingredients from the appropriate eating plan, and using recommended herbs and spices to enhance the healing.

# the digestive system
One of the main cornerstones of Ayurvedic theory and medicine is that the gastro-intestinal tract (GI) is by far the most important and crucial part of the body because it is considered to be the focal point, or the principal seat, of the doshas. Vata is formed inside the colon, pitta in the small intestine, and kapha inside the stomach. In other words, this tract has extra dimensions not recognized by traditional medicine.

## Constipation
Drink warm liquids; hot water is acceptable, but not chilled water. The best herbs for constipation are triphala and satisabgol (psyllium husks). (Do not use triphala if you are pregnant or suffering from ulcers of the GI.) Triphala is a combination of three herbal fruits, each of which has a rejuvenating effect in relation to one of the doshas. Satisabgol is a demulcent laxative. It is gentle and soothing and holds moisture in the colon, thus helping vata, which is known to be quite dry and cold. Use satisabgol with triphala; they complement each other well.

## Gas, Bloating, Colic
These symptoms are usually related to constipation. Ideally food should pass through the system in 24 hours. If it is left for much longer the process of fermentation begins, which causes a build-up of gas. The traditional herbal remedy for this is hingvastak, a mix of asafoetida, pippali, ginger, black pepper, cumin, wild celery seeds and rock salt. Another traditional remedy is a massage with brahmi oil. It restores and relaxes the nervous system.

*Eating a healthy vata diet can aid many vata problems associated with the gastro-intestinal tract.*

## Acidity/Heartburn
Sip aloe vera juice (without any citric acid added). Add fresh and dried coriander (cilantro), turmeric, saffron, coconut, fennel or peppermint to your diet. Shatavari (Asparagus racemosus), licorice (not to be used with high blood pressure or oedema) and amalaki are all used in traditional Ayurveda medicine in order to balance unwelcome levels of acidity.

## Diarrhoea
Pitta diarrhoea is generally hot, and often yellowish and foul-smelling. Diarrhoea is mainly related to pitta but can sometimes be caused by other factors, such as high toxicity (ama), stress or emotional factors. Persistent symptoms must always be dealt with by an experienced, professional physician. If you have diarrhoea, avoid eating hot spices and carefully follow the pitta plan. Eat abstemiously if at all, drinking plenty of fluids. A simple straightforward diet of rice, split mung dhal and vegetables is most suitable for the pitta dosha, taken while symptoms last.

## Persistent Hunger/Increased Appetite
In general, follow the pitta plan as outlined and use aloe vera juice as above. Increase relaxation, meditation and yoga. Also, have a long massage with brahmi oil. If strong symptoms persist, do please promptly consult your physician.

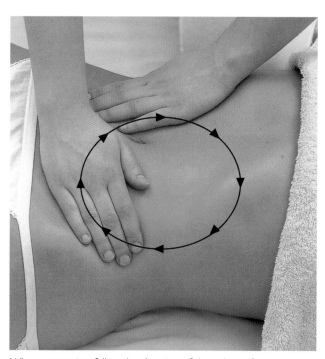

*When massaging, follow the direction of the colon – from lower left, across the abdomen, up to the right and across to the left.*

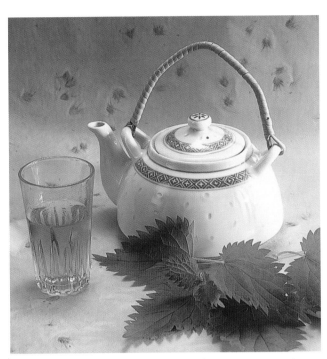

*Nettle tea is very good at balancing the digestive system and can help to alleviate pitta conditions such as diarrhoea.*

## Nausea

Nausea can quite simply be defined as the strong sensation of needing to vomit. It might not actually result in vomiting, but produces a queasy, lingering feeling that needs to be quickly relieved. It certainly is not pleasant.

Ginger and cardamom tea is often very good at calming nausea. To make it, peel and thinly slice a piece of fresh ginger, add five cardamom pods and pour boiled spring water over them. Leave to stand for about five minutes, and then stir and drink while still refreshing and hot.

Ginger is also what is known as a carminative and a stimulant. This means that it has two key abilities, first to combat any intestinal bloating, and second to speed up processes in the GI so that balance is soon restored.

During the winter and spring seasons when kapha is seasonally high, dried ginger can be blended with some boiled spring water and a little fresh honey to help keep the digestive system active and moving. This also has the excellent effect of helping to reduce the possible risk of colds, coughs and flu, and any other winter bugs that might otherwise keep you confined to the bed or house for a number of days.

Cardamom (common in southern India as well as other tropical areas, and now freely available in supermarkets) can be used for kapha and vata digestive conditions. However, it can only be used in small amounts because it can quickly aggravate pitta, or bring about a high level of pitta excess.

As with all the recommended foods, herbs and spices, the purer the quality, the more beneficial they will be. Therefore, try to buy top quality, fresh organic herbs and spices whenever it is possible. You will immediately appreciate the difference.

## The Doshas and the Gastro-intestinal Tract

### Kapha

Typical kapha conditions of the GI include poor appetite – kapha tends to be low in agni (digestive fire), which can create a slow metabolism and weight gain; nausea; a build-up of mucus, leading to colds, sinus problems, coughs and flu; and poor circulation, resulting in a build-up of toxicity (ama). Follow the kapha plan and eat plenty of hot spices, such as chilli peppers, garlic, ginger and black pepper, until the condition clears, after which you should reduce your intake of hot spices. Herbs for kapha conditions of the GI include trikatu ("three hot things"), to be taken or added to meals. This contains pippali, ginger and black pepper. You should also have plenty of vigorous exercise.

### Vata

Regular daily bowel movements are a sign of a healthy GI. Typical vata conditions of the GI include constipation, gas/flatulence, and tension – cramps or spasms, such as irritable bowel syndrome.

### Pitta

Pitta digestion tends to be fast and "burns" food. This is made worse by anger or frustration. Begin a pitta-reducing diet and eat in a calm and relaxed way. Typical pitta conditions of the gastro-intestinal tract include acidity and heartburn, symptomized by belching and acid indigestion; diarrhoea or frequent loose bowel movements, and constant hunger, accompanied by consequent irritability.

*Hot kapha dietary spices.*

# common problems
It is quite clear that the forms taken by various commonly occurring illnesses, and the appropriate remedies, will vary according to whether you have a vata, pitta or kapha dosha. The following sections therefore aim to give you individually a plan of action, setting out all the do's and do not's. Note that in the case of any persistent, or indeed serious illness, you must immediately contact a qualified professional expert.

## Insomnia
Any vata-increasing influence can contribute to your insomnia, including regular travel, stress, an irregular lifestyle, and the excessive use of stimulants such as tea and coffee. The herbs used to treat vata-based insomnia are brahmi (Centella), jatamansi, ashwagandha (Withania somnifera) and nutmeg. Any good massage using brahmi oil will also produce considerable, quickly noticed benefits.

Insomnia in the pitta dosha is brought on by anger, jealousy, frustration, fever, excess sun or heat. Follow the pitta plan, which is cooling, and take brahmi, jatamansi, bhringaraj (Eclipta alba), shatavari and aloe vera juice. Massage brahmi oil into the head and feet. Again, this is marvellously refreshing.

As kapha types like to sleep and tend to be rather sleepy and sluggish, they rarely suffer from attacks of insomnia.

## Headache/Migraine
Vata headaches cause extreme pain and are related to anxiety and tension. Relevant treatments include triphala to clear any congestion, jatamansi, brahmi and calamus.

Pitta headaches are associated with heat or burning sensations, flushed skin and a visual sensitivity to light. They are related to anger, frustration or irritability, and will be connected to the liver and gall bladder. Treatments are brahmi, turmeric and aloe vera juice. Kapha headaches are dull and heavy and can cause nausea. There may also be congestion, such as catarrh. Have a stimulating massage with minimal oil.

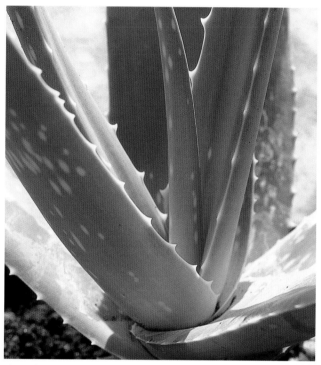
*Juice from aloe vera plants can be used to combat sleeplessness.*

*A foot massage with brahmi oil will often relieve insomnia.*

## Colds
A tendency to mucus production or catarrh/phlegm is unpleasant for the sufferer, and is usually the result of poor digestion of foods in the stomach which increases ama (toxicity) and kapha. In general, kapha is generally considered the most highly effective dosha.

Vata-type colds involve dry symptoms, such as a dry cough or dry throat. Herbs for vata coughs and colds are ginger, cumin, pippali, tulsi (holy basil, Ocimum sanctum), cloves and peppermint, licorice (not to be used with high blood pressure or oedema), shatavari and ashwagandha. Put one or two drops of sesame oil up each nostril, and then follow the vata plan until all the symptoms are seen to subside.

Pitta-type colds involve more heat, the face is usually red and there may even be a fever. The mucus is often yellow and can actually contain traces of blood. Herbs for tackling pitta coughs and colds include peppermint and various other mints, sandalwood, chrysanthemum and small quantities of tulsi (holy basil). Follow the pitta plan until your symptoms begin to subside.

*Cardamom pods are beneficial to vata-type coughs.*

Kapha colds are thick and mucusy, with a feeling of heaviness in the head and/or body. Avoid cold, damp weather and exposure to cold and damp conditions. Eliminate sugar, refined foods, meat and nuts, dairy products, bread, fats and oils from the diet and use plenty of hot spices. Drink a spiced tea of hot lemon, ginger and cinnamon with cloves or tulsi, sweetened with a little raw honey. Herbs for kapha colds are ginger, cinnamon, pippali, tulsi (holy basil), cloves and peppermint. Saunas and hot baths will help to increase the heat of the kapha person, but they should not be used in excess as this would actually increase the pitta too much. Follow the kapha plan until the symptoms subside.

## Coughs

Vata coughs are dry and irritated with very little mucus, the chief symptom being a painful cough often accompanied by a dry mouth. Herbs and spices for the vata cough include licorice (do not use this if you have high blood pressure or oedema), shatavari, ashwagandha and cardamom. Follow the vata plan until the symptoms subside.

Pitta coughs are usually associated with a lot of phlegm. The chest is congested and very uncomfortable, but the mucus cannot be brought up properly. There is often fever or heat, combined with a burning sensation in the chest or throat. High fevers should be treated by a physician, and people suffering with asthma should consult their doctor immediately if a cough or cold leads to wheezing and difficult breathing. The best herbs for pitta coughs include peppermint, tulsi (holy basil) and sandalwood. Follow the pitta plan until the symptoms have completely subsided.

With kapha coughs, the patient usually brings up lots of phlegm, and suffers a loss of appetite combined with nausea. The chest is loaded with mucus, but this may not be coughed up because the kapha individual is likely to feel tired. Treatments for kapha coughs are raw honey, lemon, cloves and chyawanprash (a herbal jam). Follow the kapha plan until the symptoms subside, increasing your intake of hot spices, and do try to use trikatu powder. Also keep warm.

## Skin Problems

These are often caused by internal conditions of toxicity (ama) and are mainly related to the pitta dosha. Vata skin problems will be dry and rough. Avoid letting the skin dry out. Herbal remedies for vata skin are triphala and satisabgol. Pitta skin problems will be red and swollen, often with a yellow head. Avoid sun, heat or hot baths, and increase your intake of salads. Follow the pitta plan and add turmeric, coriander and saffron to your diet. The remedies are manjishta (Rubia cordifolia), kutki (Picrohiza kurroa), turmeric and aloe vera juice. Kapha skin problems involve blood congestion which can cause the skin to form thick and mucusy whiteheads. Increase your level of exercise, and follow the kapha plan. Treatments should always include a small amount of calamus with some dry ginger and quantities of turmeric.

## Urinary Infections

Excess cold water, tea, coffee, and alcoholic drinks will weaken the kidneys. Salt, sugar or foods that are rich in calcium, such as dairy products or spinach, will similarly tend to weaken and toxify the kidneys. The best kidney tonic to use in Ayurveda is shilajit, a mineral-rich compound from the Himalayan mountains, but avoid it if you suffer from kidney stones. Pregnant women, children or those on medication should consult an Ayurvedic practitioner before treatment.

## Cystitis

In vata people, cystitis will tend to be less intense. Remedies are shilajit (to be avoided if you suffer from kidney stones) with bala (Sida cordifolia), ashwagandha and shatavari.

Cystitis is mainly a pitta condition because it burns and is hot. Follow the pitta plan, using plenty of coriander (cilantro) and avoiding hot spices. Remedies include aloe vera juice (not to be used in pregnancy), lime juice, coconut and sandalwood. Kapha-type cystitis is accompanied by congestion and mucus in the urinary tract. The treatments are cinnamon, trikatu combined with shilajit, gokshura and gokshurdi guggul.

*It is worth having a supply of fresh mint and other herbs to hand for many of the common Ayurvedic treatments.*

## Picture credits

*The publishers would particularly like to thank the following photographers for the use of their pictures:* Michelle Garrett, Alistair Hughes, Lucy Mason and Debbie Patterson.

*Thanks also to the following libraries for supplying pictures:* A-Z Botanical Collection Ltd: 35BL; 47TR; 52BL; 60BL; 61BL, BR; 62BR; 63TL; 65TM. Bruce Coleman Collection: 62BM; 63TM; 64BM. Frank Lane Photographic Agency: 39BM. Garden & Wildlife Matters: 38TL; 59BM. The Garden Picture Library: 36BL, TR; 38TM; 39BR; 63BL. Images Colour Library: 74B. Harry Smith Collection: 53BL; 61TM; 64TL, TR; 65BM. Tony Stone Images: 35BR; 68T, B, 71B; 72B; 78B; 82B.